I0117811

Bodywork for Babies
Parent's Companion Guidebook

Susan Vaughan Kratz

Published by Ten16 Press, an imprint of Orange Hat
Publishing, 2024

PB ISBN: 9781645387824

Copyrighted © 2024 by Susan Vaughan Kratz
All Rights Reserved
Bodywork for Babies Parent's Companion Guidebook
Written by Susan Vaughan Kratz

This publication and all contents within may not be
reproduced or transmitted in any part or in its entirety
without the written permission of the author.

Ten | 16
PRESS

orangehatpublishing.com

For my daughter Emily, who inspired me to leave no stone unturned

Medical Disclaimer

The contents of this book are intended for educational purposes for health and wellness conditions. This book is not a substitute for medical advice, diagnosis, or treatment. This book does not include complete or exhaustive content applicable to any specific medical condition. The contents of this book can, however, be used in conjunction with other bodywork endeavors and shared with your providers for mutual care of your baby.

Liability

The reader assumes full responsibility for using the information found within this book. The reader agrees that the author and publisher are not responsible for any claim, loss, or damage resulting from using this information by you or any user.

Seek professional guidance if the contents of this book need further explanation, clarification, or demonstration.

Copyright

No contents within this manuscript may be reproduced without permission. All copyrightable text, graphics, design, and selection of information are based upon the author's clinical experience and are exclusive rights of Susan Vaughan Kratz unless otherwise noted.

Photographs are the author's property or have been licensed for use from Shutterstock.

There are evidenced-based therapies....
and then there is the real world.

This book is about the real world.

This book offers real solutions
that have helped real babies and real families.

This book offers techniques that can assist with soothing and easing a
baby's everyday struggles that can be stressful for families.

This book is written for every parent who
believed in the changes their babies revealed
in bodywork sessions, and trusted the process of
self-correction with assistance
of trained hands.

Table of Contents

Introduction

The *Bodywork for Babies Parent's Companion Guidebook* was written in response to requests for an instruction manual teaching parents how to soothe their babies. Lactation consultants, midwives, and pediatric practitioners praised the idea of such a resource.

This book's contents are designed to empower parents with a deeper understanding of the anatomical reasons behind their babies' everyday struggles. Several practical bodywork techniques are included and are easy to implement by following the basic instructions for each. Based on years of performing bodywork on infants and witnessing the positive changes, I teach these same techniques to many parents on how they can help their baby at home.

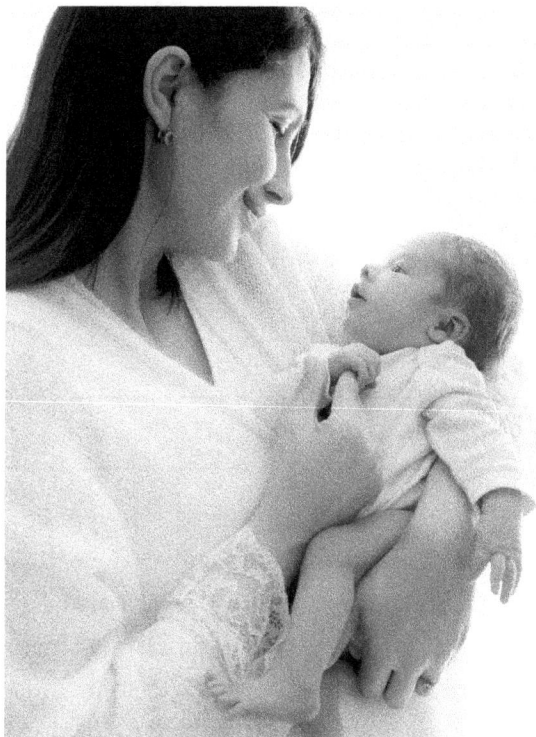

> This book recognizes the needs of parents of newborns worried by issues:
>
> - You're not alone when struggling to help your baby's body adjust
>
> - These stresses & strains can be identified & helped by trained hands
>
> and
>
> - These body tensions can also be helped by your gentle hands and a simple roadmap

My first book, *Bodywork for Babies,* was written to support pediatric therapists in the learning curve of CranioSacral Therapy, visceral manipulation, myofascial release, lymphatic and lympho-fascial mobilization, and other soft tissue methods. Many relieved parents also bought that book with excitement that some answers to their babies' discomforts were defined. And simple treatments made available.

This book is a companion guide specifically designed as a home program. The opinions and suggestions are based on the knowledge gained in my 40-year occupational therapy practice and over 25,000 client encounters. These pages honor thousands of babies that guided my hands in gentle ways to locate and ease:

- Body strains left over from being held tight in the womb and birthing
- Breastfeeding struggles and management of tongue ties
- Colic; reflux; constipation; digestive un-ease
- Irritability; self-regulation; sensory modulation
- Torticollis and misshapen heads

These common issues are frequently a problem of compressed organs and the surrounding connective tissues. As a result, organs, blood vessels, and lymphatic pathways can have added resistance against fluid flow and optimal function. Muscles and soft bones can be torqued, pulled or twisted, which can keep a baby in a constant or near-constant state of stress. Also, soft tissues can draw in protectively (retraction) when the circulatory and nervous systems are stressed.

It is a false assumption that babies "grow out" of these issues by waiting to mature or by solely spending time on their bellies. The old notion of "wait and see" is becoming replaced by sound osteopathic and bodywork wisdom. The knowledge was learned by many practitioners worldwide spending extensive amounts of time listening to body tissues. The listening is done with our hands. These simple and gentle methods often change things quickly.

Bodywork for Babies helps establish health and wellness as a good start in life

---

In the first few weeks of life's journey, the baby's primary job is to self-regulate physical functions. Behaviors like colic and prolonged fussiness are not normal, though very common. Though not every baby (or family) suffers through colic, it means through body communication that things are not as good as they could be. That something needs attention. As the fussy baby grows, and if these problems don't resolve, other behaviors of stress or self-regulation can develop. When a child's stress stays high, family stress increases.

Retained compressions and body strains from being in the womb, or from the birthing process held in your baby's body, may not always correct from their own stretches and movements. They do try to self-correct such tensions, but it is common that many babies have some area that could use some assistance. Their communication to us through their behaviors is their attempt to self-correct tissues.

Body tension is one expression of the autonomic nervous system. The primary indication of increased body tension is caused by blood vessel walls constricting (vasoconstriction). In my twenty-five years of applying bodywork to infants, I have treated only five babies that didn't present with some type of compression or tension issue. Common issues include compressed heads and necks, retained pressure into face structures and nerves to the mouth and tongue, distorted rib cages and pulls at the diaphragm, umbilical cord remnant under the belly button, bands of fascia that are taut, shortened muscles in the neck, shoulders, or hips, among other things.

A sustained hug calms and relaxes us in the same way as swaddling, and the chief effect is the relaxation of the blood vessel walls (vasodilation). Swaddling is calming because of the deep pressure, which is similar to the womb experience. Deep pressure helps the body turn off stress and relaxes us into the rest and digest state (parasympathetic state). Body parts can reverse the protective retraction then. *Bodywork for Babies* primarily addresses the autonomic nervous system state of your infant. Bodywork training guides us practitioners to locate what deep body part most needs a hug, the attention for help in relaxing and dilating surrounding blood vessels.

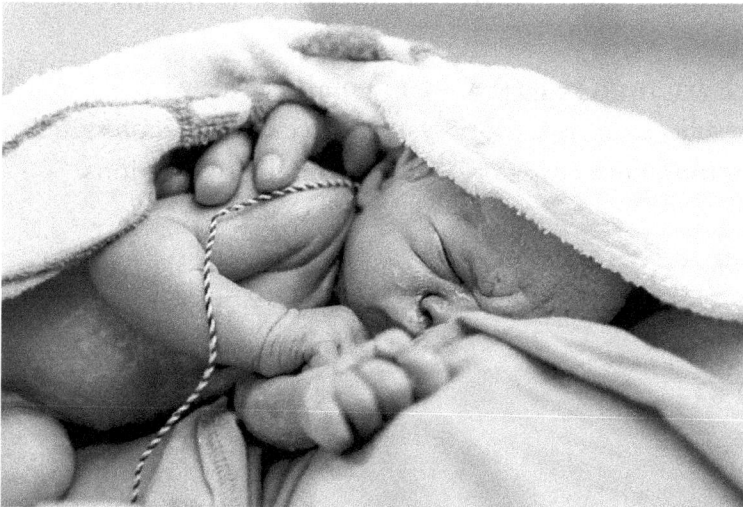

One's occupation is any task that occupies your time. For babies their main occupational job duty is self-regulation, followed by learning to eat, interact with the environment through their senses, move their bodies, bond emotionally with caregivers, and develop play skills. Any retracted tissues in the body can interfere with your baby maturing these tasks efficiently, especially during the fourth trimester. The fourth trimester is approximately twelve weeks after birth when your baby adjusts to life as a separate being.

Bodywork for Babies can help your baby do their job of self-correcting body, nerves, organs, and soft tissues to master these jobs:

1. **Optimize breathing:** expand rib cage; mobilize lungs and heart space; activate muscles between ribs; ensure a flexible respiratory diaphragm.

2. **Self-regulation**: activate and balance the autonomic nervous system continuum; adjust circulatory system and blood vessel response to changes in temperature and oxygen levels in the blood; react and respond to various sensory events; recover from the reaction to sensory events without sustained stress; self-soothe when comfort measures are given (holding, rocking, swaddling); begin to regulate digestive system (from mouth to anus).

3. **Get ready to master gravity**: lift head and upper body uniformly; stretch out body limbs and torso in various positions; tolerate and be active in tummy time; roll equally both directions; stabilize head and eyes to gain a sense of midline.

4. **Get ready to learn from senses:** react/respond/recover within five primary conscious and five primary subconscious sensory systems; free compressions around sensory organs and nerves; learn from both conscious and subconscious sensations.

Conscious	Subconscious
* Seeing	* Body movement sense
* Hearing	(kinesthesia)
* Smelling	* Muscle/joint pressure sense
* Tasting	(proprioception)
* Touching	* Organ sensation
* Head movement sense	(interoception)
(vestibular)	* Emotion sensation
	(enteroception)

5. **Oral function in readiness of best nutritive and non-nutritive sucking**. Reflexes which support the early learning of skills which are needed to master nutritive and non-nutritive sucking, include: coordinate breathing & swallowing, midline control of head on shoulders for best swallowing; manage a large amount of sensory information; freedom to move tongue fully; maximal jaw movement; control of lips; press tongue fully into roof of the mouth; pull tongue backward to create a vacuum draw on nipple.

Parents instinctually know when their baby is not comfortable or when they are holding tension and stress in their body. However, they may not have a frame of reference of what to do about it. Some common signs from your baby may include:

- Scrunched up face; looks grumpy
- Grunts excessively; pulls stomach inward; tight belly
- Whole body doesn't seem to eat, digest, or eliminate with ease
- Back is stiff when being picked up and held; arches backward uncomfortably
- Body and spine is still in a forward C-curve by the end of the first month
- Dislikes being in a car seat or being on their stomach
- Baby's body doesn't seem to relax
- Chin touches chest; ears touch shoulders
- Head tips to one side
- Favors turning head or looks to one side when lying down
- Deep creases in neck; difficult to clean the neck skin
- Performance difference between sides when breastfeeding
- Retracted or compressed lower jaw; sunken-in lower lip; tight upper lip
- Can't open mouth wide enough to cover nipple; or opens unevenly

This parent's companion for *Bodywork for Babies* includes the most frequently taught methods in our work with families. To include all the methods considered "bodywork" in one book would be impossible. This collection is the most frequently used, and the ones that consistently help babies get to a place of self-correction of stresses and strains held in their bodies. We've used these methods routinely to help colic, constipation, reflux, breastfeeding challenges, torticollis and head reshaping, and tongue tie management.

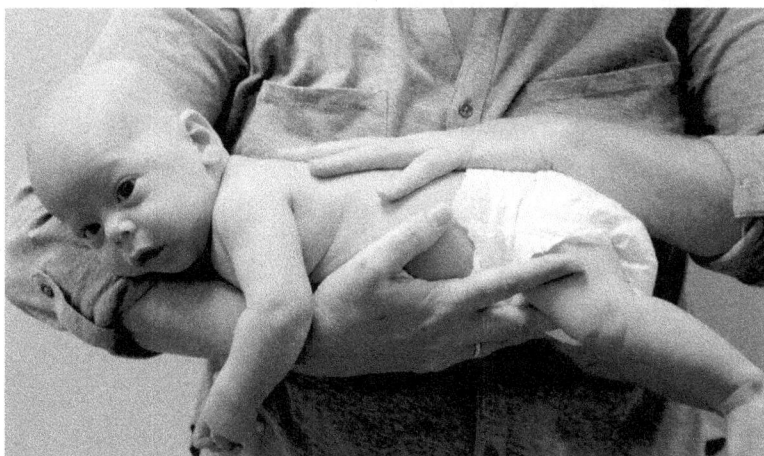

Body Communications

Before and **After** one session of *Bodywork for Babies*. Your parental instincts likely tell you body tension in the left photo is problematic, and in the right, more desirable.

Before

After

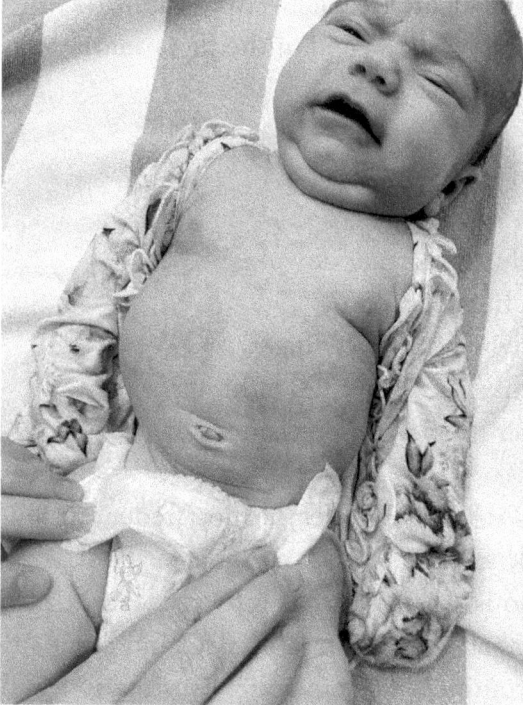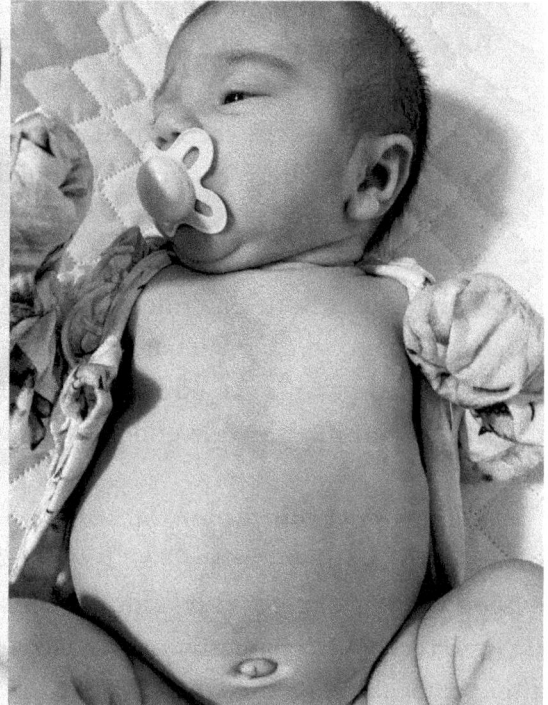

Baby's body in the left photo might be communicating this:

- I have compressed nerves in my face or neck
- Organs in my tummy are too tight or weak to move food & waste
- My spine has tension when I'm curved in my car seat
- Even though my baby bones are soft, they may be compressed
- My shock-absorbing fascia can't work out the birthing strains
- There may be a hidden torticollis from tissues pulling in my neck
- My jaw may be pushed backward on my face
- I'm stuck in fight-flight because of emotions I'm having or sensing
- My umbilical cord is pulled inward, see this in the belly button

Issues in the Tissues

The book's contents will help parents understand the anatomical reasons for common struggles. Strains in the tissues can become functional and behavioral concerns.

To help dispel any sense of feeling overwhelmed if this information is new to you, let's break things down into manageable chunks of material:

1. Tension throughout body, stiff back and tight neck

2. Colic, reflux, [baby] constipation, grunting to defecate

3. Breastfeeding challenges: latch, tongue tie, tight mouths, fatigue, coordination

4. Self-regulation and sensory modulation, fussiness, self-soothing, sleep performance

5. Torticollis, distorted bodies, misshapen heads, and asymmetrical faces

6. Common issues with arms, legs, and ears

1. Tension throughout body, stiff back and neck

Tension can be held anywhere…. neck, shoulders, hips, knees, throat, and head. Even the face and mouth can hold tension, often due to compressed nerves and fascia. Babies frequently arch their backs during the first few months of life as a natural way to stretch out of fetal position. The critical thing to remember is how long your baby stays tense and whether they can actually get to a relaxed state with these body parts.

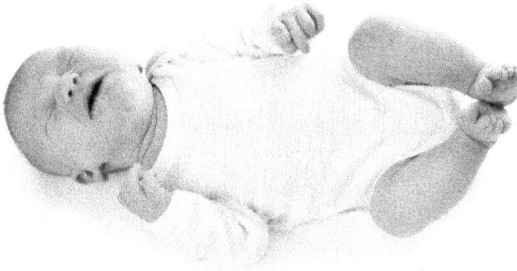

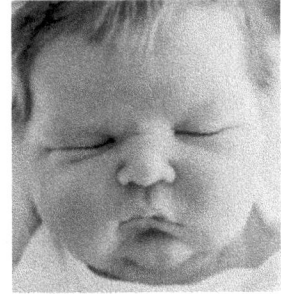

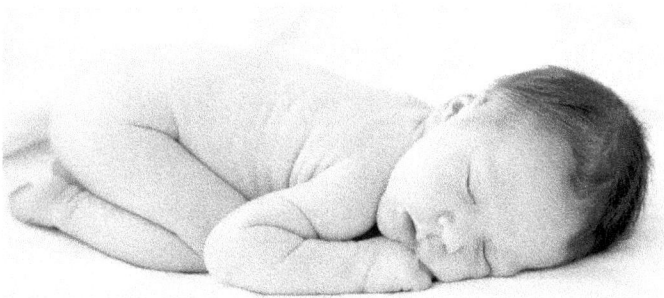

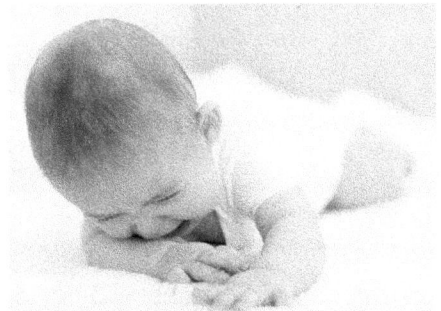

Tissue tension can sometimes cause crying and frustration, but not always. Baby's hips and legs have been bent for several weeks in the womb, leading to shortened and tight muscles in the pelvis and knees. Connective tissues have shock-absorbing properties, and the strains of being curled in the womb or from the birthing process can be retained in these tissues. Such tissue restrictions can pull on the lower digestive organs, creating behavioral stress.

What can't be seen with the eyes, can be felt with the hands. With practice, compressed or retracted organs can be felt and compared for tone: (liver, stomach, intestines, major blood vessels, and mass of blood vessels especially in lungs and between intestines). There are basically two states of being: tight or loose. Tense or relaxed state. Bodywork eases and can balance tensions in just a few sessions.

2. Colic, baby constipation, reflux, grunting to defecate

Tell someone, "My baby has colic," and watch their universal reaction. A baby that cannot soothe itself can make a strong man weak in the knees, and the most resilient woman melt into tears. An inconsolable baby can lead people to lose a sense of reason and rational thought. Finding immediate solutions to alleviate such discomforts is the collective caring thing to do.

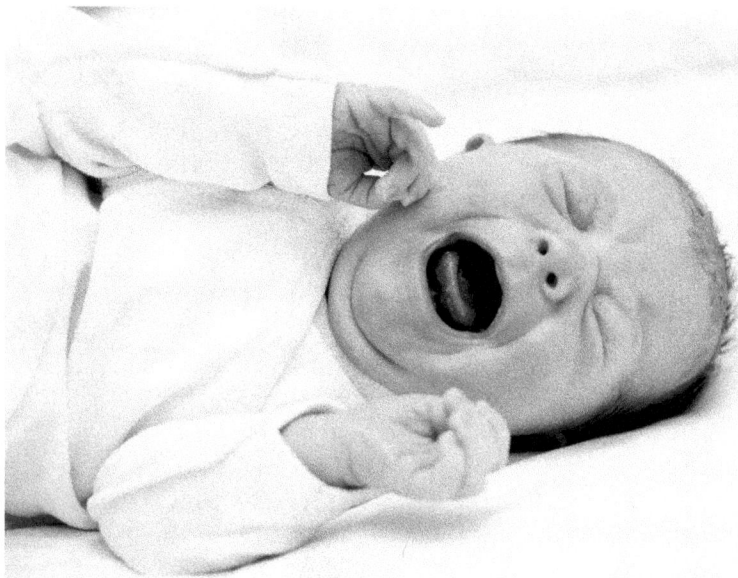

Colic is frequent, prolonged, and intense crying or fussiness in an otherwise healthy baby. It has been described in some professional books to last anywhere from three to eighteen months. This distressing behavior seems to occur for no apparent reason and is an expression of dysregulation of organs and the autonomic nervous system. Baby's behaviors of grunting, crying, flexing or arching body, and demanding intense distractions are attempts to adjust and cope with internal discomfort. For hands trained to listen in bodywork, babies have consistently communicated to us what many of the reasons could be.

Colic communicates discomfort of immature digestive tract walls and possibly tight sphincters (valves spaced throughout the tract). Reflux communicates tension or torsion at the top of the stomach.

Colic communicates tension at the lower part of the stomach and upper small intestines. Baby constipation is generally not the same as adult constipation. Immature walls of intestines may not be strong enough to move solid waste through the system.

The walls can have resistance imposed into the system from pulls of the umbilical cord and intestine migration during fetal development. Neighboring structures when tight, such as the respiratory diaphragm or the hip muscles, can also pull on these organs. Added resistance interferes with the ease of food and waste moving through the intestinal tract. The liver and the bile duct can have increased tension from similar types of strains, especially the remnants of the umbilical cord buried behind the belly button. These tensions can be present without causing a full-blown medical problem.

The most common techniques we have witnessed to help relieve symptoms of colic and excessive fussiness include releasing tissue restrictions around: the ribs, the respiratory diaphragm, the entire length of the digestive tract and its surrounding connective tissues, the digestive sphincters, and the hip flexor muscles. Sometimes, relief is found after a baby passes gas, has a bowel movement, or achieves a significant burp. Trapped gas is likely swallowed air during feedings and prolonged crying. Tense organs and weak organ walls contribute to trapping air bubbles.

Fussiness may be related to any of these resistances within the digestive tract or from compressed nerves or tissue in the neck, head, or face. If the birth was particularly challenging or traumatic, consider that the soft bones of the skull may hold compressions from the forces encountered during birthing. This is a common finding in babies who continually fuss daily, week after week when no other medical issue can be identified.

When to call the doctor:

Try bodywork from a pediatric therapist, such as an occupational or physical therapist or chiropractor with bodywork skills and training. When excessive crying is not resolved with attempts at relaxing the body organs and muscles discussed in this book, seek consultation with a pediatrician or gastroenterologist.

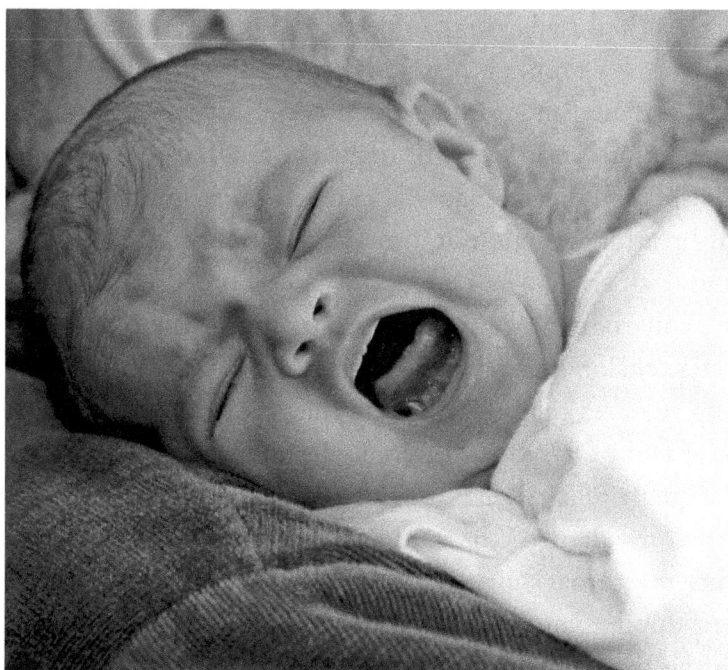

3. Breastfeeding Challenges
(latch, tongue tie, tight mouths, fatigue, regulation)

Understanding that successful breastfeeding is a whole-body endeavor can be empowering. Feeding is not just about the mouth but a process that starts in the oral cavity and moves through the chest, rib cage, and respiratory coordination.

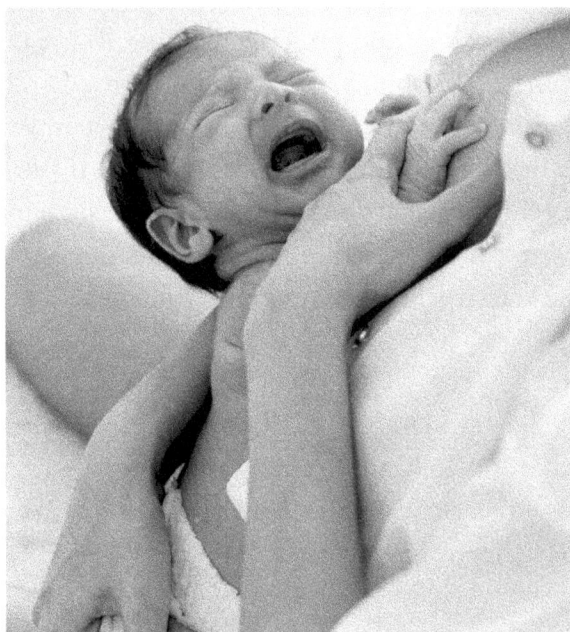

First, the chest and belly need to be free of core tension so that breathing is at its best. Feeding involves a rapid pattern of suck-swallow-breathe in rhythm. The breath timing can be affected if anything torques the rib cage, lungs, or blood vessel masses. Body tightness can make fatigue set in faster or make the feeding process take longer. Thus, an underappreciated aspect of breastfeeding is efficient breathing.

Inefficient breathing, while not a medical crisis, is a subtle quality of movement issue. Shoulder and neck tension can affect the ease of breathing because the upper lungs rest just under the collarbones. Many structures around the front of the neck and upper rib cage can transfer tension into breathing.

Swallowing requires many body parts that project to the middle of the body be free of tension or absent of tissue restrictions. A good sense of midline balance develops when the body is equally relaxed on both sides of the body. The nose, chest, belly button, and hips should readily align to the middle. This allows swallowing to occur without straining to protect the throat's airway in each suck-swallow-breath cycle. To highlight this, try turning or tipping your head sideways and swallow. Notice that tension? How difficult would eating be with tension in your throat?

In addition, the jaw has numerous tissues attached down the front of the neck, projecting into the shoulders. Mouths that can't open wide enough to cover the breast nipple often have muscle and fascia tension in the jaw, lips and cheeks. The tongue is attached to muscles in front of the neck and inside the curve of the jaw. When the jaw is tight, often pushed backward and upward, the tongue can be pulled backward into the mouth. This stress pattern occurs because increased tension demands more airway protection, interfering with swallowing ease. Once the tension is released in the jaw, face, neck, and shoulders, the suck-swallow-breath pattern usually improves as the reflexive feeding can proceed unhindered.

The increased awareness of tongue ties has increased the demand for bodywork before and after a surgical release of tight tissues. Connective tissue bands connect the tongue to the body's core down the entire length to the toes. Several issues, not just the frenum tissue, can contribute to the lack of tongue movement.

It's also important to remember that breastfeeding success is not solely dependent on you or your baby. Families need and deserve support and resources when breastfeeding doesn't happen automatically. All babies who are struggling to feed can benefit from some bodywork. Parents having a little Bodywork knowledge can bring a sense of hope and reassurance.

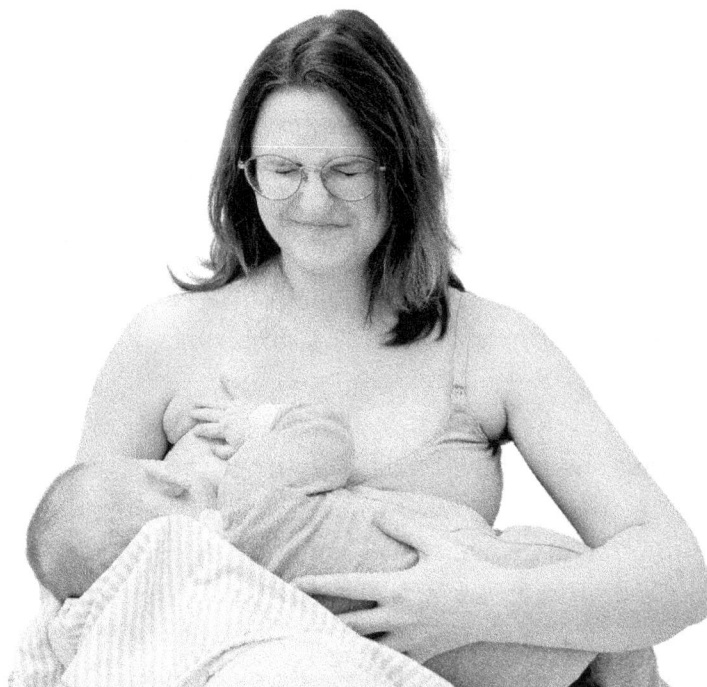

Tongue tie

A tongue tie (known as ankyloglossia) is an abnormally tight band of tissue that attaches the underside of the tongue to the oral floor. A tie is not an isolated piece of tissue. It has become evident through the research of fascia that a tongue tie is related to whole-body fascia. These bands are part of the "soft skeleton" that creates body form and suspension support for organs and muscles.

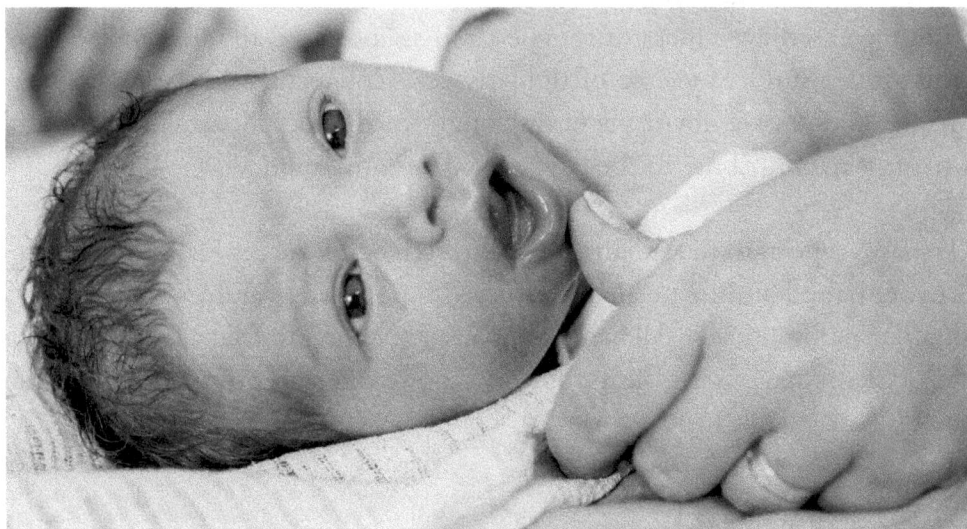

Tongue tie affects about 5-13% of all newborns. Boys are three times more likely diagnosed than girls, and ties tend to run in families. Ties are a common cause of breastfeeding problems, and when corrected, breastfeeding typically improves. Ties affect tongue movements and can interfere with speaking, eating, and dental alignment. Symptoms include distinct tongue appearance, tongue can't lift or extend past lower gum line, and a lack pressure into the roof of the mouth. But it is common to have none of these symptoms and still have tethered tissues. This is known as a functional tie. If left untreated, ties can become related to future problems such as eating intolerances, hyperreactive gag responses, stress behaviors around food, speech impediments, and even obstructed breathing such as sleep apnea.

The baby's tongue should fill 90% of the space in the mouth, resting and pushing into the roof. The normal pressure from sucking during feeding and on pacifiers help flatten the palate into a functional surface. Tongue ties keep the tongue from elevating fully to press into the roof of the mouth. If the hard palate (roof of the mouth) is higher arched, it often means the tongue can't fully elevate and give adequate force to shape the soft bones during infancy. Pressure into the roof also calms and regulates the nervous system. Reflexive sucking of the mouth is an automatic soothing agent.

The tongue acts as a natural palate expander when it has the range of motion and control to press upward during sucking (both nutritive and non-nutritive sucking). The hard palate is a surface for the tongue to work off, but it is also the floor of the nose. Small nasal passageways can be part of high-bubble palates. Hyper nasal sound production or unintelligible speech production can be related to these high, "bubble" palates. Mouth breathing disorders, troubled airways, and sleep disorders can also co-occur.

Many different professionals have developed therapeutic interventions for tongue ties and oral dysfunction. Myofunctional therapists arose from a collaboration between speech therapy and dental care providers specializing in the mouth's function. Originally designed for ages 4 and older, myofunctional therapy has evolved to include younger children. Dentists or orthodontists who address palates for bone and teeth alignment, offering dental expander if needed.

Pediatric therapists specializing in feeding and development who also practice bodywork address tongue ties from the whole-body perspective, not just working inside the mouth. Early childhood therapists qualified for feeding therapy who address tongue ties and oral function are most commonly occupational therapy and/or speech-language pathologists. Qualified lactation consultants may become specialists in tongue-tie management related to breastfeeding. Remember, tongue-tie management is a subspecialty interest, and no one profession requires training to practice and treat this condition. Additional training is required beyond a degree. Parents should interview resources or search for a local preferred provider list.

Whole-body assessment is best practice if your baby has a suspected tongue tie.

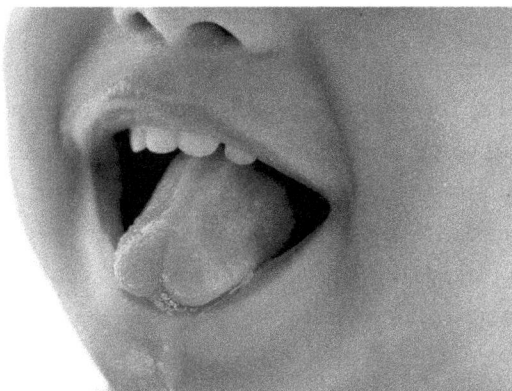

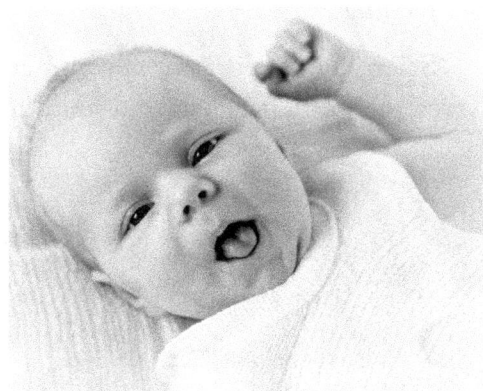

Appearance suggesting a tongue tie:

- Line of tight tissue in the middle of tongue, tight attachment to tongue floor appearance
- Tongue is flat or squared when tongue comes forward (should be pointed or round)
- A heart-shaped or notched tip of the tongue
- Tongue doesn't stick outward or come forward beyond the lips

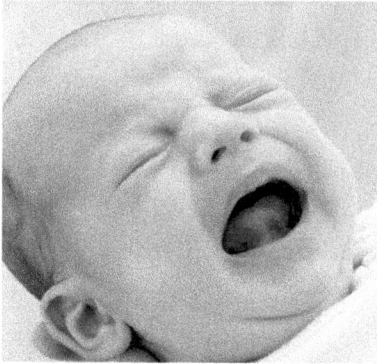

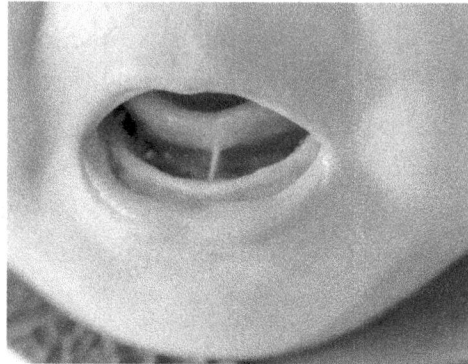

Functional movements suggesting a tongue tie:

- Tongue movement: can't lift fully to hard palate (roof of mouth); or move side to side; -
- Tongue doesn't fully curl around a nipple or your finger
- Tongue is weak or struggles to draw backwards to transfer milk towards throat
- Presence of a high-arched hard palate
- Poor quality of latch on breast nipple during feedings
- Clicking of tongue or gulping air during feedings
- Does not manage a coordinated suck on a pacifier
- Fussiness from lack of efficient suck to self-sooth or not deep enough from feedings

Scientific support for recommendations on managing tongue ties is growing. However, there still needs to be a solid care plan for every person. It has been determined that tongue appearance must be considered equally to functional movement. The methods of surgical repair range from cutting to releasing tight tissue with a cold laser. Lactation consultants and speech therapists have established a place as tongue-tie management team members. What still needs consideration is the timing and amount of bodywork and fascial release. Parents should have access to any of these professionals for thorough evaluation and treatment planning, including parents' point of view with equal measure. Each individual case is unique.

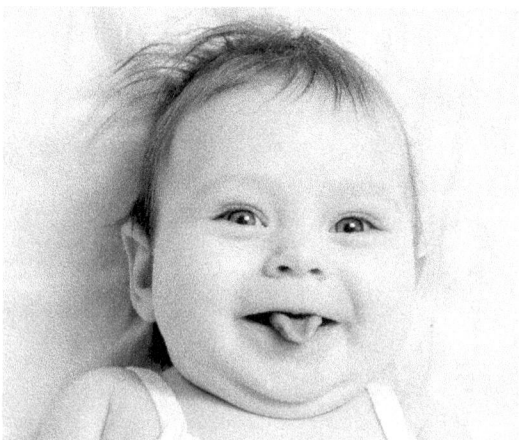

4. Self-regulation and Sensory Modulation
(fussiness, self-soothing, sleep performance)

Body tension can turn into behavioral challenges. A significant nerve that influences digestion and helps humans relax is located where the bottom of the head meets the top of the neck. When this nerve (vagal nerve) retains compression or is torqued and strained by surrounding bone, digestive organs can shut down. As a result, the autonomic nervous system is kept in a state of chronic distress, especially when you hold your baby sideways to challenge the neck supporting itself.

As a parent, you can play a crucial role in ensuring your baby's vagal nerve is in its "happy place." If the head still holds compressive forces into the neck and shoulders caused by birthing, the neck appears short or crunched, and the vagal nerve is likely compressed. This can also lead to tension in the jaw, throat, neck, and shoulders, contributing to fussiness, irritability, and inefficient feeding. Knowing this empowers you to take proactive steps to help your baby's tissue relax & soften.

Understanding your baby's behavior and function doesn't have to be complicated. In fact, it's quite simple. Nerves, organs, and blood vessels that are otherwise healthy have only two terms to communicate to us:

Structures are either:
Tight or loose; tense or relaxed

Babies love it when we know how to listen with our hands to locate tension in body parts. They love it more when your hands become confident in your ability to soothe the tension away.

Learning to soothe tensions is gained from straightforward communication from body tissues as your baby shows you where to work. Tight areas or organs means the sympathetic (fight-flight-freeze; stressed) state is activated, causing constricted vessels. Things tighten up, and fluids, foods, and fecal matter don't flow as well because tension increases resistance. In a state of tightness, reactions to sensory information can be alarming and distressing. On the other hand, loose means: the area or organ is in the parasympathetic (rest and digest, relaxed) state. Things soften and relax so fluids, foods, and fecal matter flow easily from space to space, decreasing resistance and improving blood flow. In this state, babies are more likely to respond well to sensory input and not startle.

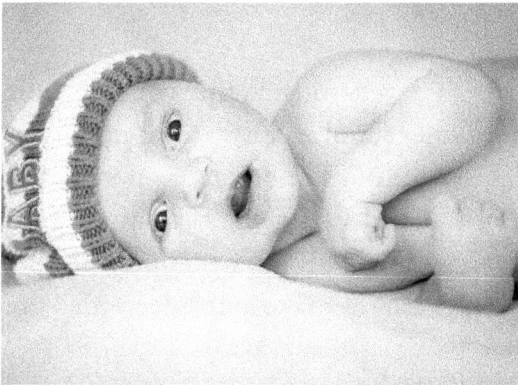

5. Torticollis, misshapen head, distorted body and face

As a watchful parent, you would likely notice any prominent head tipping or twisting to one side (torticollis). It is commonly described as only wanting to look or turn the head in one direction. Babies can't really make such a choice. When torticollis exists, there is nearly always a connective tissue undertone. Rather than a baby wanting to look to one side, their head is pulled toward the soft tissue restriction(s). The head can be tipped sideways in a straight direction, torqued in a rotation, or a combination of both.

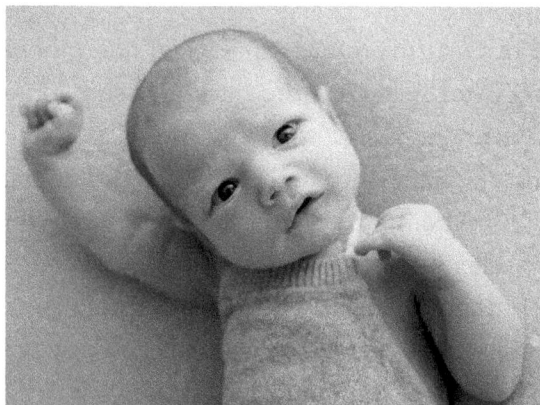

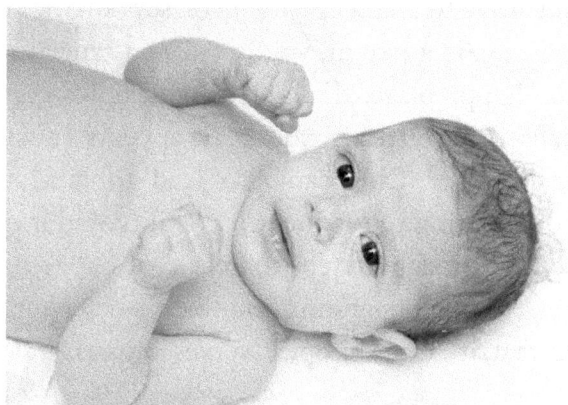

Torticollis, whether congenital or acquired, can develop inside the womb or from mechanical forces and strains during birth. It can also occur after birth from prolonged back lying with the head turned to one side. The severity of the condition can vary. However, it's crucial to remember that early detection and treatment can significantly improve the outcome. This potential for improvement can instill hope and optimism in you as a proactive parent, knowing that you have the power to make a positive difference in your child's health.

Old assumptions suggest that torticollis is caused by short neck muscles. However, the wisdom gained from whole-body bodywork reveals that rarely are just the neck muscles involved. Many tilted necks are often pseudo-torticollis. Twists and turns in the rib cage, internal organs, and even fascia down the body into the hips can wrench the head and neck in a direction that prevents the head from correcting itself towards the middle. When the neck is bent or rotated at an odd angle, the symmetrical balance of the head and face can also be affected.

Left untreated, torticollis can lead to unequal head control, limited eye tracking, eye teaming problems, less arm reaching, unequal rolling to both sides, balance and posture issues, crawling performance, and future coordination concerns.

Torticollis in infancy should ALWAYS be evaluated and treated by an experienced and qualified pediatric professional. A pediatric occupational therapist or physical therapist is also suitable for developmental and movement assessment and treatment. A therapist with both bodywork method training and a specialty in development can be a perfect team leader to ensure all aspects of torticollis become resolved. A pediatric chiropractic evaluation is also warranted to ensure the neck bones are not displaced (subluxation).

It is a condition that a baby does not often grow out of. Traditional stretching exercises can be challenging for parents and babies to tolerate. *Bodywork for Babies'* unique combination of methods are innovative ways that can speed up the self-correction of the body. Bodywork is best addressed before six months of age, after which time babies desire to be more mobile and may have a trickier time tolerating staying still for bodywork.

Mishappen Head

The bones of your baby's head are growing within a bowl of dense connective tissues. A thick layer of fascia (dura mater) just under the skull bones surrounds the brain and protects it very well. The bones will protect the insides of the skull once the hardening (ossification) process completes itself. The timeline on which this bone maturation occurs differs for each bone. The most important thing to consider during infancy is that many of the skull bones are in segments. These pieces of growing bone grow within the fascia bowl.

The spaces between the bone segments (soft spots) will fill in as the bony plates grow and reach the margins of the neighboring bones. There are several soft spots, though the more prominent ones commonly get the most attention. Bones can become out of alignment where edges of growing bone can heave into the soft spot. These can be felt as bumps or ridges on the head. This situation is most commonly a result of the forces encountered during birthing.

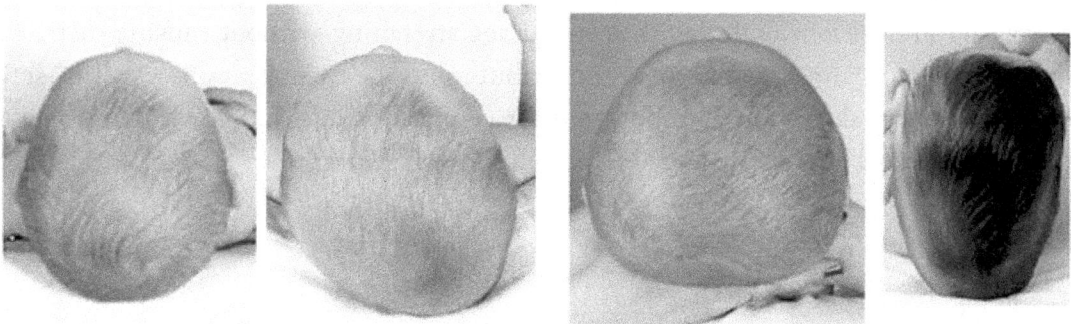

The "molding" of your baby's head during birth can result in a cone-shaped, elongated, or asymmetrically shaped head. Research on MRI scans shows that a baby's head will remold itself within days of birth. Suppose the head does not remold itself on its own. In that case, it may indicate that the forces of birthing or positioning in the womb are still held within the shock-absorbing tissues of the skull. This is where bodywork methods, especially CranioSacral Therapy, are a perfect match for helping. There is no scientific evidence that misshapen heads cause any harm to the brain. Still, clinical practice suggests that specific cranial nerves are vulnerable to being strained or pinched when the head bones are not freed from restricted soft tissues.

Babies can also develop flat spots on their heads due to immature neck muscles that can't entirely turn for several weeks as a newborn. This phenomenon has long been recognized as a result of the international back-to-sleep campaign as a measure to reduce the risk of sudden infant deaths. When a baby lies only on one side for an extended period, the risk of a flat spot developing increases. This happens because the bones in the baby's head are still very soft. (The condition of a misshapen head is called plagiocephaly.) Mild flat spots can naturally go away when babies spend equal or more awake time on their tummies, on your chest, or from caregiver babywearing. Changing positions for resting, sleeping, and playtime can help to remold the head shape and prevent flat spots.

Eustachian tubes can be compressed, eye socket differences in size and form can affect the eye muscles, or flattened bones can push other bones out of alignment. Whenever there is a bump or ridge on the crown of the head, one bone will most likely override the neighboring bone. Much clinical evidence has shown that the gentle method of CranioSacral Therapy can correct those bony overrides. So, more than appearances and esthetics, head shape contributes to the overall health and wellness of the head and face and the nerves that weave between the bones.

Parents, your role in the treatment of torticollis or a misshapen head is crucial. By engaging in positions and play that encourage stretching without causing distress to both you and your baby, you are actively contributing to the treatment process. This active involvement can make you feel empowered for your baby's health, knowing that you are not just a bystander but a key player in your child's well-being.

6. Common issues with arms, legs, and ears

Babies clench their fists for different reasons. A reflexive grasp, which starts in utero, prepares hands and fingers for movement. Pressure into the palm of the hands can be how your baby seeks comfort and security. Hands can also reflect internal states of tension. Tight fists can mean hunger, feeling cold, or tension in some organs. One way to know this is to watch what the hands do once your baby is warmed and has a full tummy.

During playful waking hours, your baby's hands will likely relax with outstretched fingers. Grasping skills develop as the fingers unfurl. After the fourth month, the hands should not be fisted very often, indicating circulatory, muscle, and nervous system maturation.

When to be concerned is when the hands are fisted most of the time with little time being relaxed. Bodywork methods can help you as a parent understand the reasons why fisting persists and assist those palms and fingers into comfortable positions.

The arms and legs can be scrunched because the long nerves off the spinal cord travel through a lot of flesh that can hold tension. Their immature shoulder, elbow, hip, and knee muscles are indeed shortened, and they don't have the strength to stretch for several weeks. Sometimes, groups of muscles and the connective tissues surrounding them are restricted so that organs and blood vessels in the area hold increased stress. This can contribute to behaviors of fussiness and difficulty settling.

All of the long nerves end in the hands, feet, and ears. The ends of the nerves rest within muscle, organs, and other structures and retract in a state of alarm or stress. It is possible to help relax nerves, the nerve endings, and the body parts they control with simple and easy-to-apply application of bodywork methods to these three areas. Once you learn them and discover their effectiveness, you might use them frequently in play and interacting with your baby. Anything that you as a parent can do to relax all the body parts that react to stress and tension sets you both up for a lifetime of being adaptable and resilient, better at non-verbal communication, and better able to cope with stress. Bodywork is a primary way your baby communicates their needs and your hands listen and try to meet those needs. Your baby will then grow knowing that they can trust you to address sources of stress. This builds a foundation of resiliency for emotional and physical health and wellness.

Analyze Your Baby's Body

Body symmetry can be appreciated with some guidance on what to look for. We notice when sides are equal and intersections are balanced. Use these grid lines to train your eye to monitor your baby's body positions after birth.

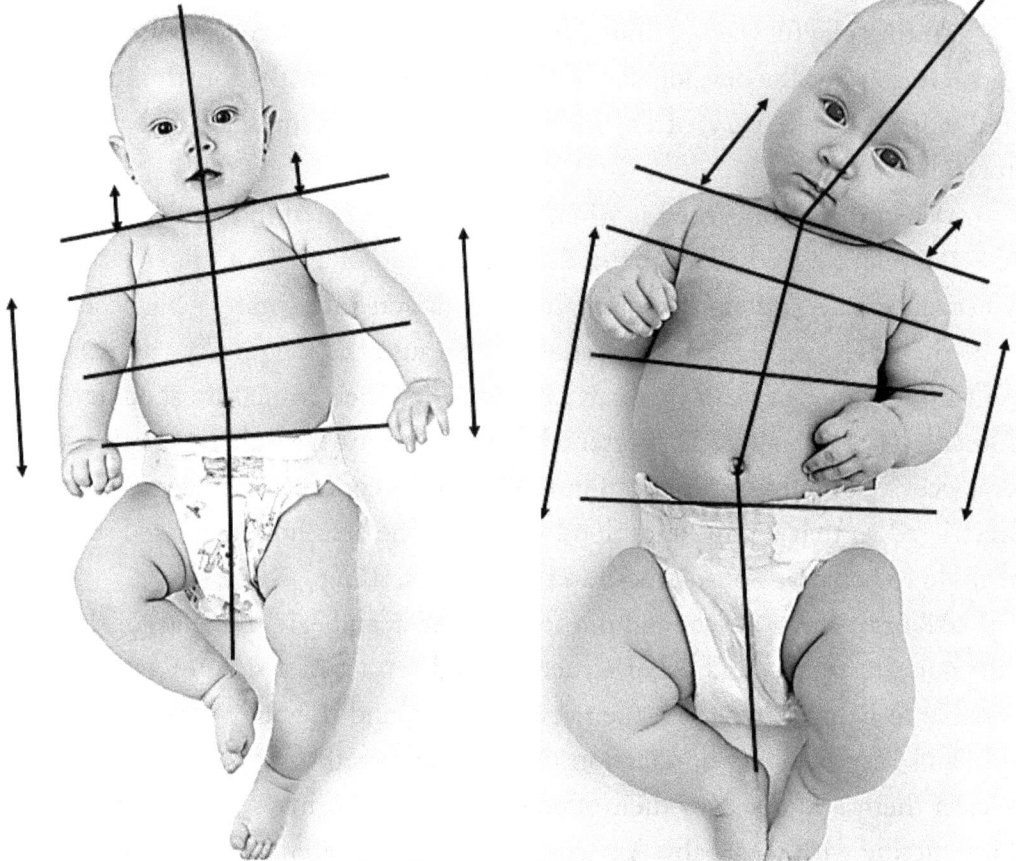

Reference Lines

Central lines:
Throat to top of head
Belly button to throat
Belly button to tailbone
Sides: armpits to hips
Ears to shoulders

Horizontal lines:
Tips of shoulders
Nipple line
Lowest rib point
Top point of hip bones

Face Symmetry and Ear Alignment

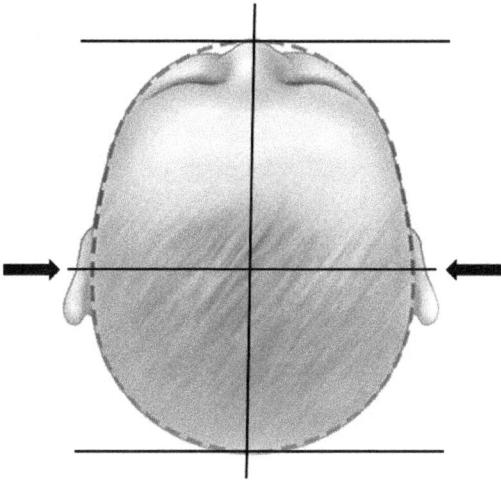

This grid helps your compare the halves of the front and the back of your baby's head. You can appreciate ear alignment by looking at the top of the head. Any flat spots or shifting can be noted, and your comparisons can be made from week to week, month to month. If change is not happening, you will have information to share with any pediatric professional you are seeking services from.

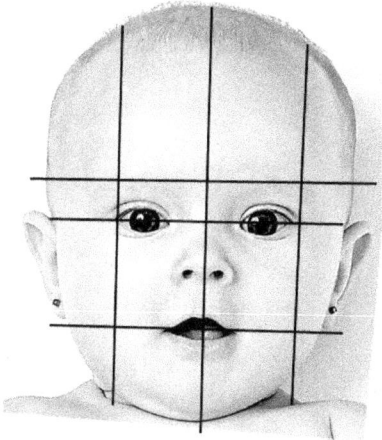

Symmetry of facial features can also reflect head bone and tissue distortions and any plagiocephaly patterns. Eye shape and size, the level of ears, the level of mouth corners, and the vertical lines of the nose and eye corners are targets. Grid lines help train your eye as you inspect the face

Like many other infant interventions, early diagnosis and treatment are more effective when head or face misshaping is addressed as soon as possible. Early treatment can shorten the duration of intervention. Based upon changes we have observed in helping babies' heads to self-correct in remolding, *Bodywork for Babies* offers an alternative and complimentary intervention to a cranial helmet.

Simplified Anatomy

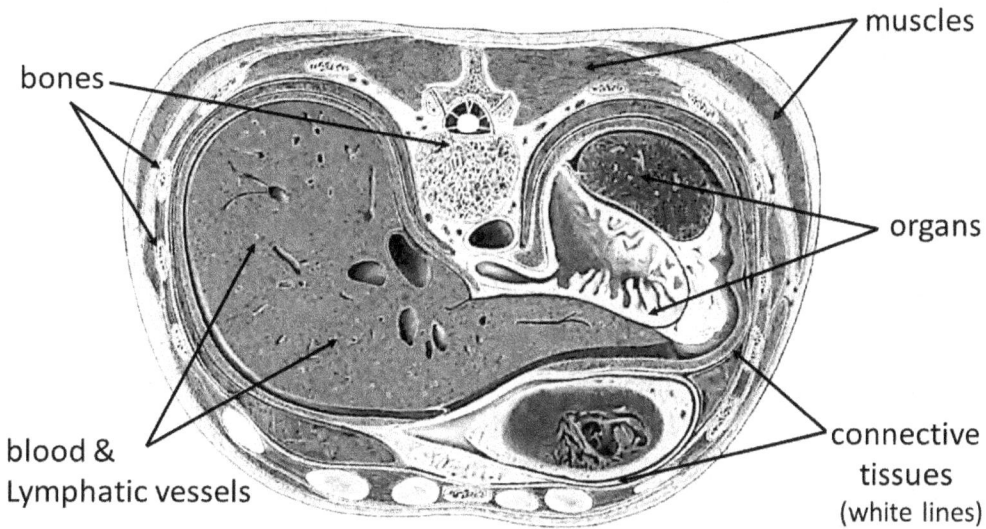

bones

muscles

organs

blood & Lymphatic vessels

connective tissues (white lines)

The Visible Human Project of the National Library of Medicine, Public Domain

Inside the body, there are lots of organs and structures packed tightly together. Look at the above illustration of the cross-section through the human abdominal cavity. You'll see bones, muscles, and organs; look even closer and see blood, lymph vessels, and white lines depicting connective tissues. Look under a microscope and find millions of arteries, veins, and tiny nerves. What you don't see in this illustration is much open space. Structures are packed closely for efficiency. Open space is a waste of real estate in the body. But organs and parts must slide against their neighbors to be calm and happy. Birthing and positions held in the womb can push organs and connective tissues together, creating a state of stress that doesn't change until the structures decompress. It is a false assumption that all babies simply grow out of compressed states.

It is challenging to learn anatomy and remember the multitude of names of body parts; it can be overwhelming. When it comes to therapy, we are bound by the educational system that stresses the accuracy in naming of things. Abiding by that expectation only stresses out the person, especially when it comes time to feel for a structure with our hands. However, when it comes to helping another person, it is not necessary to know the names of all the body parts.

Consider the idea that the body is actually quite simple. After all, your baby started as two cells joining together, multiplying, and then specializing to become organs with different functions. Despite specializing, cells have relatively simple reactions when it comes to stress. They tighten, or they loosen within the autonomic nervous system state. Muscles get the blame (or credit) when tension and stress are felt in the body. This is true, but it does not reflect the whole truth. This belief discounts the effect of microscopic reactions on all structures in the body. Connective tissues are shock absorbers of physical events, which means fascia contracts or retracts. Blood vessels and nerves tighten from any threat or force, and the structures they serve tighten if some or all remain retracted or stressed. Moving bones apart to free up nerves by overpowering any tension by force seems to be our natural bias. Chiropractic and physical medicine methods have a long history of trying to get muscles to relax by working the larger parts. The kind of force dictating our approach to the adult body is the absolute wrong way to approach the body of a baby. Perhaps this bias explains why many professionals may be scared to work with infants.

The manual therapy methods of *Bodywork for Babies* take a reverse approach. We believe (from experience) that a baby's muscles, organs, and even bones can decompress themselves given enough time under helping hands. Muscles, organs, and nerves will tighten as a homeostatic reaction to preserve the cellular world and meet the demands of fluid around cells. When tissues has tension, resistance to flow increases and movement and exchange of fluids reduce. The way we hold in *Bodywork for Babies* allows for fluids to seep back into tissue it was compressed out of due to mechanical stressors. When fluids seep back into connective tissue layers, blood vessels expand and relax, then muscles and organs relax. Only then are nerves freed from compression.

The secret to CranioSacral, visceral, and lymphatic methods is waiting for fluids to permeate through tissue layers, which soften tension to all structures underneath our hands. We apply these methods with a universal therapeutic touch. Most tension is the fight-flight or freeze response of cells, organs walls, and connective tissue from the stress and forces entering the body. Like any hug from one person to another, a calming and soothing effect can happen if a touch feels "just right." A microscopic yet non-invasive "hug" can describe the hands-on method described in the following pages. This is how we help babies in their daily struggles. The key is knowing exactly where to place your hands, how to touch when you place them, and how long to hold them there.

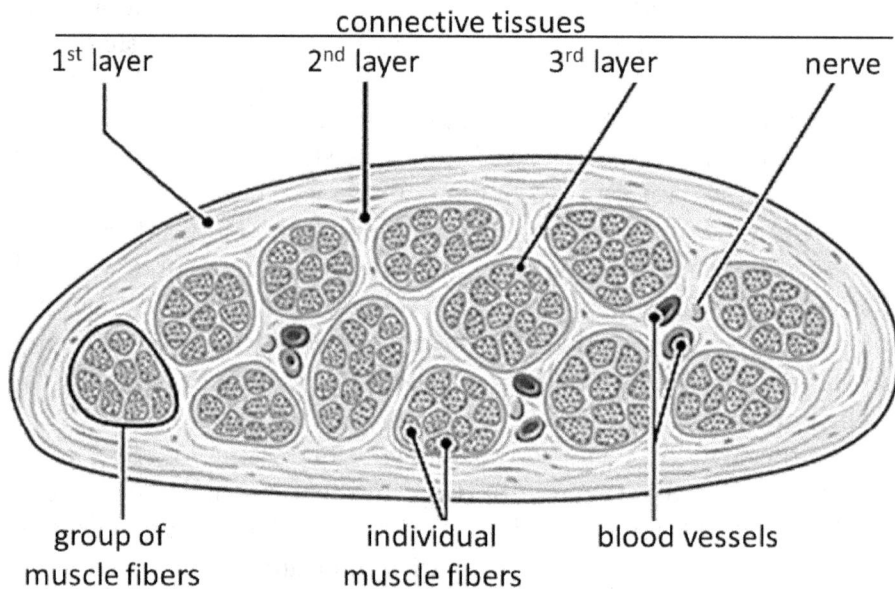

Visualize the cross section of a typical muscle. Layers of connective tissue (fascia) binds strands of muscle filaments, woven with blood and lymphatic vessels. All these structures hold a high content of fluids. Helping the tension ease, releases these fluids and puts the areas into a relaxed (parasympathetic) state.

The *Just Right Hold*

- Different Kinds of Touch
- Teaching Your Hands
- Practicing the *Just Right Hold*
- How Not to be Afraid of the *Just Right Hold*

Different Kinds of Touch

Touch is crucial for healthy human relationships. Tiny brains develop meaning about the things they touch and about stuff and people that touch them. Research and ancient wisdom have shown that skin-to-skin touch soothes and reduces fussiness, promotes sleep, improves digestion, helps weight gain, and improves general well-being for both a caregiver and a young baby. Skin contact regulates a baby's temperature, heart rate, and breathing better than alone in an isolated crib. Emotional attachments are forged for life as a result of bonding through touch. When doing bodywork, consider two distinctly different ways to touch your baby's skin:

MOVING TOUCH

NON-MOVING TOUCH

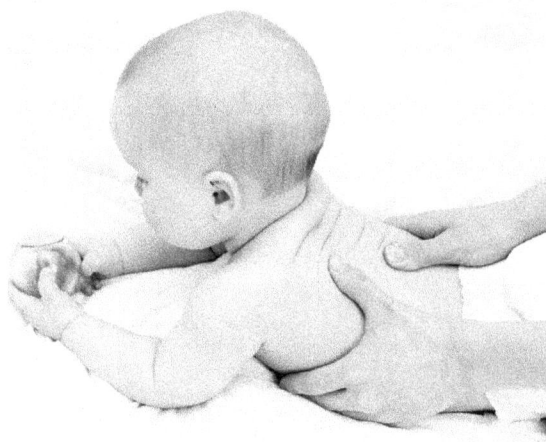

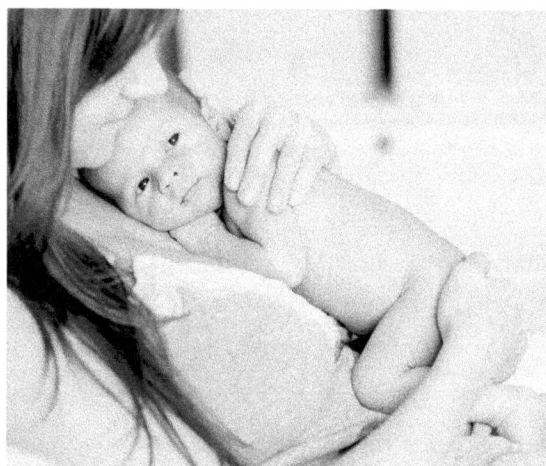

Moving touch (rubbing skin) is more stimulating and alerting. Infant massage is an example, and it is valuable for engaging and bonding with your baby. Most babies find it playful and usually react positively. When done with your baby's reactions in mind, infant massage is a "just right" input to the sensory systems, as long as it does not cause overload or stress. Stress from too much touch can look like over-excitement, fussiness, or even shutting down into sleep.

Non-moving touch (NOT rubbing skin) is calming because it resembles womb pressure. Those long months in the womb were one long embrace, so a steady type of touch input is very familiar to a baby's system. Examples of non-moving touch are: skin-to-skin body contact, swaddling, and body wearing. Staying in contact with what is underneath the skin's surface, using non-moving touch, is a critical element of the bodywork methods described in this book.

Teaching Your Hands

The moment you place your hands on your baby, you have an effect on their body. The smallest blood vessels, nerves, and fluid spaces around the cells react to your therapeutic touch. The energy from your hands will affect every single structure under the skin, all the way to bone and organs. This has been proven with sophisticated equipment, so trust that you can do therapeutic touch simply by being a living, breathing person. The loving care you match with your touch will be your intention. Trust that your baby's tissues and cells respond to the mindfulness of your touch. Science has proven that even babies can sense your intentions.

Dr. John E. Upledger, DO, OMM (father of modern-day CranioSacral Therapy), is credited for bringing this manual therapy into therapists' hands over forty years ago. He made waves with his osteopathic medicine colleagues when he publicly announced that a person need not be a doctor to practice this method. A good bodyworker needs only an understanding of anatomy and physiology and skills of approaching the client with a loving heart and pure intentions. I believe Dr. Upledger's teachings offer the *just right touch [and hold]* to help your baby›s body self-correct from the strains and compressions of birthing.

As loving and caring parents, you can learn this knowledge to the limits of your interests and confidence levels. Learning some basic anatomy of your baby and some simple manual techniques can help you get through rough times when colic, constipation, and reflux can be stressful. You can learn how to release tension and tone by understanding where to place gentle hands at precise points. You can learn how to help your baby's body parts decompress from birth and aid in the self-correction of head remolding and reflexive stretching.

When wanting to lend aid, we humans are biased towards assuming the best way to help is to massage or rub. The *just right touch* is not about poking or prodding. It is a stillness in the *holding* of your hands. We must remember that moving touch is stimulating and alerting but can be alarming if too much pressure or movement is used. Pressure or touch input that is too invasive can make tight structures even tighter because the internal organs and vessels react protectively by withdrawing as a turtle pulls into its shell or a sea anemone retracts its tentacles.

Ultimately, Baby expresses preferences for types of touch, either moving or non-moving, and communicates which they favor at any moment of time.

This book....
- ...encourages you as a parent to trust your baby's ability to communicate just where their body needs help.
- ...gives you a road map for hand placement and guidance for success.
- ...augments your knowledge but doesn't replace professional care if needed.
- ...offers help for those without local community resources.
- ...provides tips for finding a qualified pediatric practitioner.

Practicing the *Just Right Hold*

You instinctively know how to gently touch your infant, which is an excellent beginning for learning *Bodywork for Babies*. The *just right hold* requires your hands to be non-moving. This turns your hands into «listening hands» that can better find areas of deeper tension. Moving hands would miss these subtle signals. Instead of "doing things to" to your baby's back, arms, or belly, non-moving hands do things "with" your baby's own control. The power of change thus is given over to your baby and their physical abilities, instead of you feeling responsible for doing the fixing. This guide will teach you how to trust your baby's self-corrections. We call this help "holding space." The hardest part of learning this way of bodywork is waiting, and trusting in your baby's power over their own body at the tissue level. Remember, patience and using the right kind of touch are key to your baby's relaxation.

When holding still on an area of tension or tightness, your hands provide a gentle acupressure that allows time for your baby's self-corrective nature of the autonomic nervous system to kick in. This leads to small expansion of organs and blood vessels. Muscles relax when blood vessels relax. (Prodding hands can increase tension in organs and blood vessels). Your baby's nervous system communicates internal tension to your listening hands, and you'll be amazed at how well your baby can express their needs. Your hands remaining still, present, and patient, create a safe space for your baby to unwind and release deep tensions. It's important to practice and develop a belief in this process.

Here are a few ideas to help further your learning of the *just right hold:*

IDEA #1:

The touch begins with hands placed on a body part like a lily pad resting on water. The lily pad responds by doing nothing if the water is still, but then reacts to any movement or direction in the water flows. As tissues relax, you might feel a sensation of movement under your hands. Trust that you will feel tissue move under your still hands. This is how your baby's tissues relax as blood vessels dilate and fluids flow.

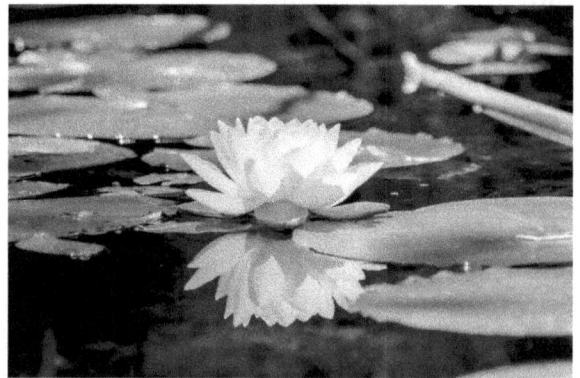

Practice thinking that your hands are like lily pad

IDEA #2

The *just right hold* waits for the tissues to lead the session. The concept of holding a cold stick of butter while maintaining the pressure of a lily pad is helpful to keep in mind. Holding butter long enough with the warmth of your hands will help soften the structure. Your baby's organs and muscles will relax the same way. This may sound absurd, but it is not. This hold allows time for the nerves to release under their own power. You just need to be patient enough and trust that this will happen. Trust me, it will.

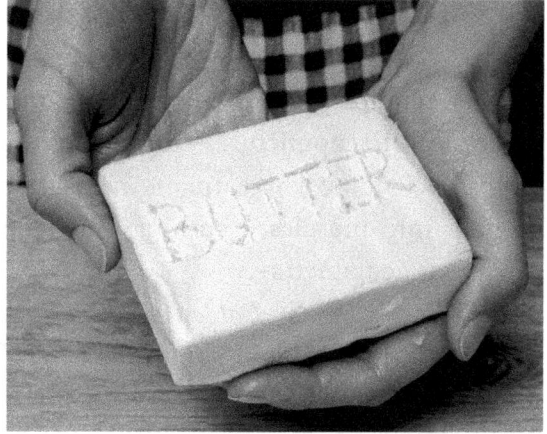

IDEA #3

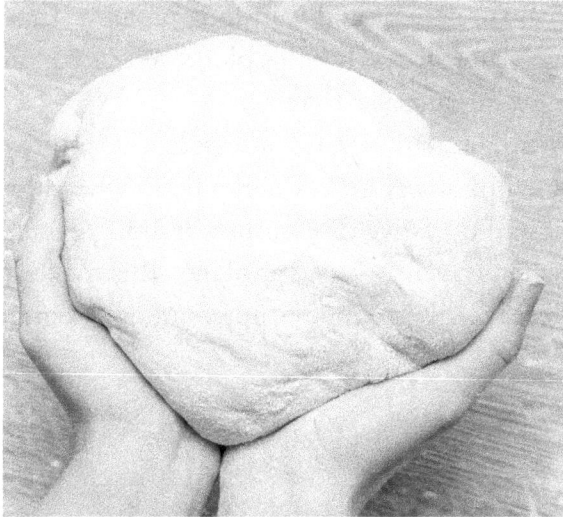

Imagine holding a large ball of bread dough, watching it react to the yeast and rise. This is akin to the final stage of helping babies self-correct. Just as we gently stretch the dough to aid its rise, body parts will naturally stretch and expand from a state of tension to softening. Your baby is leading this process, causing these changes to occur. Your hands, in a state of focused intention, remain still to receive messages from their body, then add the slightest stretch when the tissues respond.

These ideas are unique to the methods used in Bodywork for Babies. Whereas methods that move, force, or touch with pressure can create tension within the body as organs and blood vessels retract for protection from too much input. We hold the body with still hands to get the tissue communication, and we add a gentle stretch to tissues when the body says it's time.

You cannot hurt your baby if you do bodywork with these 3 ideas in mind

A Word About Acupressure

Acupressure has been used for centuries in different cultures. Based on the principles of acupuncture, acupressure does not need the use of needles to be effective. Trigger points are where fingers massage specific spots, and some versions involve rigorous digging into muscles. Learning trigger point locations can be as extensive a learning process as acupuncture.

Bodywork for Babies is less concerned teaching parents what pressure points correspond to specific organs or nerves. We simplified things based on real experiences for ease of application, removing the mystery. Rather than rely upon complicated acupuncture point maps or reflexology charts, we merely feel for tense spots with gentle thumbs. Tender, listening hands find these spots.

One a tension site is felt, apply gentle sustained pressure until the tight spot releases, just like applying gentle pressure (like to a cold stick of butter). You will be using the *just right hold* with your thumb or fingertips. Tissues will soften, relax, and become supple under your touch contact if you're patient and wait long enough. That is the straightforward explanation of how acupressure works. It helps blood vessels running throughout a muscle dilate and expand, promoting muscles to relax.

Helping blood flow reduces pain, inflammation, and stress levels, improves digestion and circulation, and even boosts the immune system. Energy flows when blood flows. Acupressure can help relieve fussiness and digestive discomfort, draining ears and sinuses, and even relieve inner ear pressure when traveling on an airplane. This makes for calmer, sleepier babies. Your little one can feel their best when acupressure is integrated into daily life.

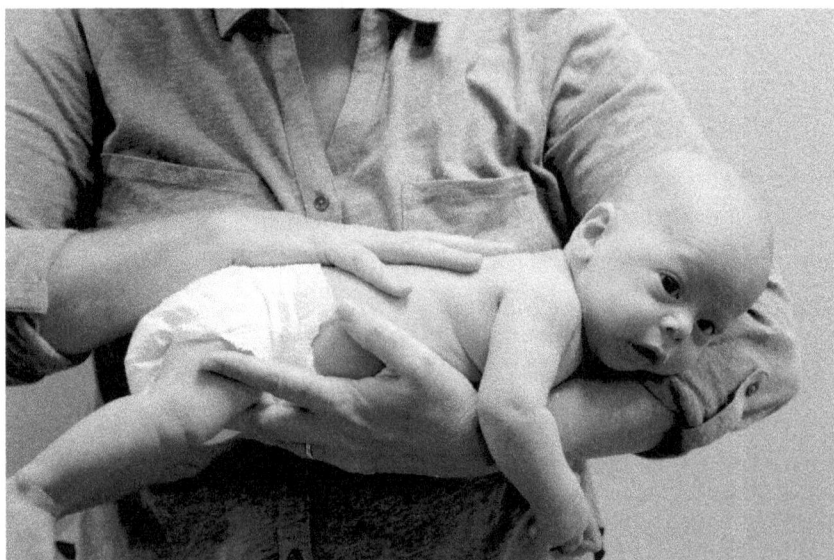

How not to be afraid using the *Just Right Hold*

Don't apply any force

Don't use your hands to squeeze, manipulate, or compress

Lay hands on a targeted body part as light as lily pads lay on water

Listen with fingertips to the tone and tension of what is under your hand

Wait, wait, wait for tension to begin to soften and relax the way cold butter begins to soften under the touch of your warm hands; be patient and wait long enough for this to happen

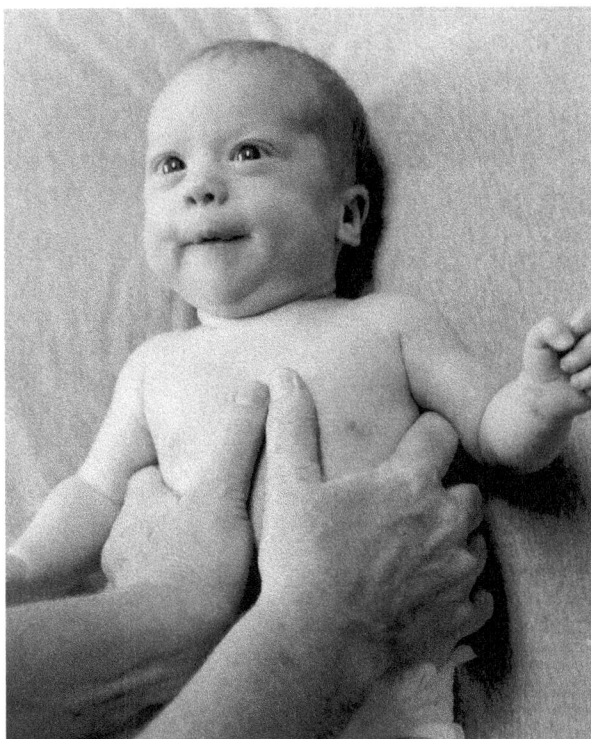

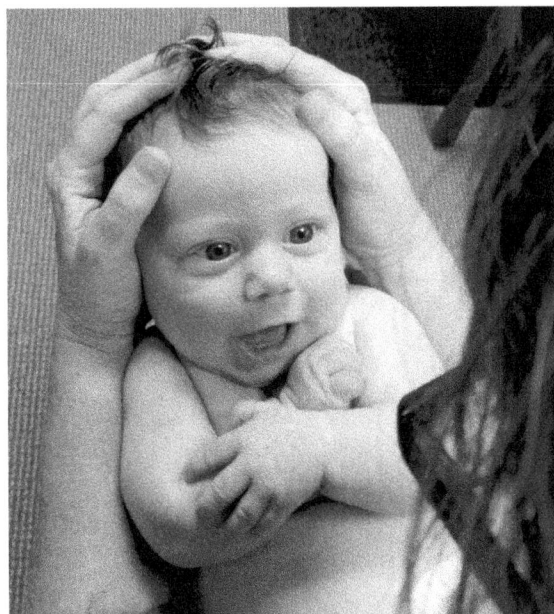

You already know how to touch your baby gently and lovingly. Now you'll have a guide to touch intentionally with the purpose of using your hands as listening tools to "soften" the problem areas and allow your baby to release their own tensions at the cellular level. Being on the right spot is the key. Work at believing that your hands can learn this simple method.

Bodywork Techniques

The history of the *just right hold* comes from the long-held knowledge of the osteopathic and bodywork professions. The goal is to help you as a parent to become empowered by information about gentle, non-invasive touch so that you can become your baby's best advocate. These techniques are designed to guide you into a journey of learning what your baby wants you to know about their own body, what they have gone through, or where they need a little help. Let your baby inform your hands. You will both become more empowered by this information and feel less helpless and frustrated.

Bodywork techniques in the next pages are organized by sections of the body:

- Chest / Neck / Back   p. 36-45
- Tummy   p. 46-54
- Arms /Legs /Ears   p. 55-59
- Head / Neck   p. 60-65
- Face / Mouth   p. 66-70

Several techniques can be used to address more than one problem. Some techniques help specific problems. Practice and see what you're successful at helping your baby's self-correction from birthing and in utero strains.

These ideas are not meant to replace professional help. Please reach out to local pediatric practitioners or therapists (See resource websites on p. 78-79).

Use this book in conjunction with any help a professional may offer. Take this book with you to any appointment and share ideas with them. Work together with your local pediatric practitioner who is well-trained in any of the bodywork methods discussed in this book.

Use the *Just Right Hold* (See pp. 27-33) for each technique discussed

A combination of:
1. Gentle touch like a lily pad resting on top of water
2. Warm & caring touch that can melt butter when you hold it long enough
3. Reacting to subtle tissue movements and applying a very slight stretch like you would react to rising bread dough in your hands

---

CHEST / NECK / BACK

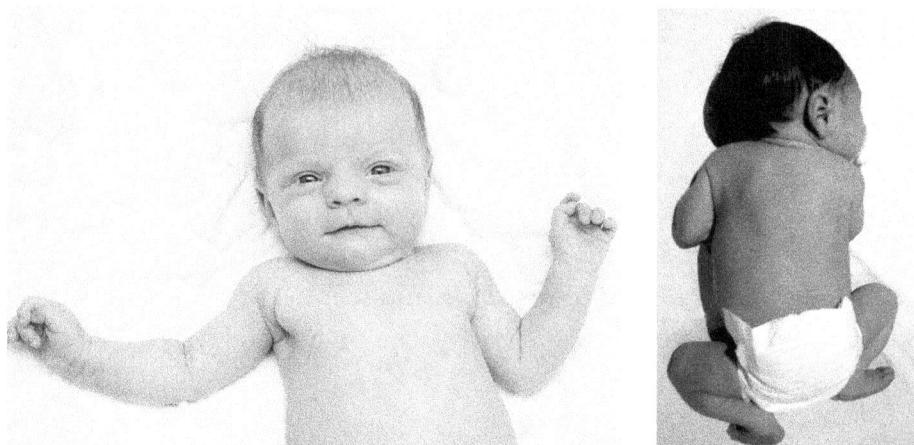

Look at your baby's rib cage on front and back sides and note its shape. The lower ribs usually flare outward and become narrow towards the shoulders. This angle is because of weak muscles between the rib bones. During the first few months, they belly-breathe using only the diaphragm to inhale and exhale. You'll see their tummies moving up and down with breaths. The little muscles between ribs will eventually mature for full expansive breathing, which takes several months. The dozens of tiny muscles between and surrounding the ribs are activated with crying, laughing, guppy pose, arm stretches, rolling, and during tummy time.

The ease of lung expansion needs to be coordinated with breaths during [breast] feeding. This can be hindered if the rib cage is drawn in tightly. The narrowing of the upper ribs can be pulled tightly inward, causing deeply furrowed armpits. Other tissues can pull or torque the whole rib cage, which determines the flexibility of tissues surrounding the lungs. These strains are commonly related to the head being pushed into the neck and shoulders from birth. In addition, tightness can come from fascia bands and remnant strains in the umbilical cords coming up from the belly button.

The rib cage can be twisted by fascia underneath the skin and where the diaphragm attaches above the abdominal organs. This is often caused by positioning tightness in the womb. Such fascia twists can create torticollis or keep babies dysregulated because each breath, though mild, may have a structural challenge. Fussy, irritable babies commonly have tightness or twists in the rib cage. Breastfeeding challenges can also be a result of a ribcage that lacks the flexibility that allows for quick breaths between sucking and swallowing.

Chest / rib cage DO NOT massage. DO NOT move your hands.

The *just right hold* over the rib cage is a perfect place to start practicing bodywork on your baby. This can be performed when your baby is lying on their back, on the tummy, being held in your arms, or lying on your chest. Hold the entire rib cage with wide-spread fingers and hands resting like lily pads upon the water. Listen with the sensations from your hands to the shape of the rib cage and notice how it expands with each tiny breath. Sit with this hand position for several minutes and several breathing cycles. Feel for any tension under your hands. Your baby will likely begin to self-correct as you're learning what the ribs want you to know. Wait for a butter-is-melting feeling.

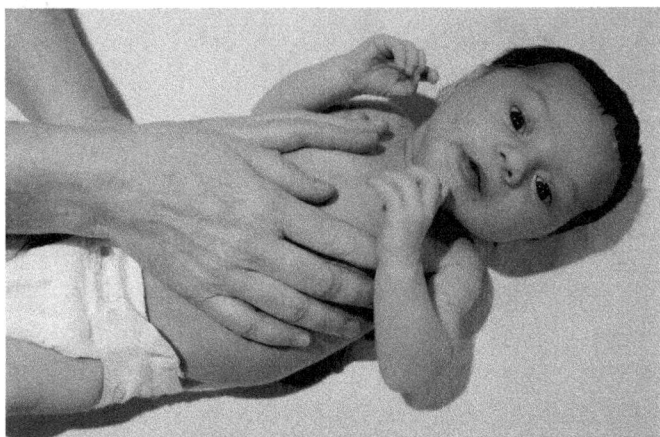

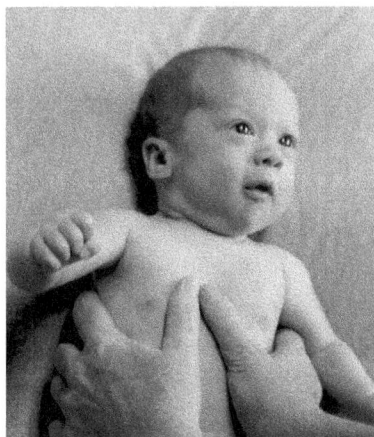

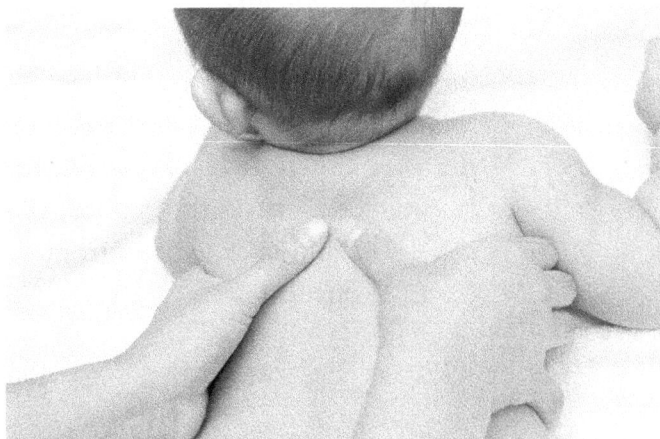

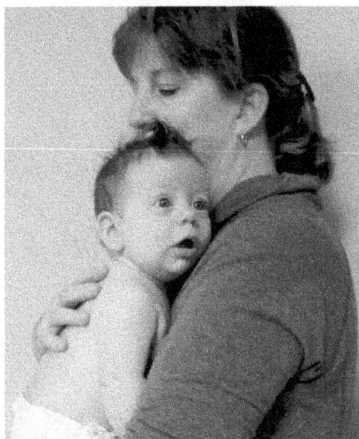

Continue to hold the ribs and interact with your baby's torso the way you would holding a rising mound of bread dough. The tissues surrounding the ribs, the lungs and heart, and the diaphragm will continue to soften and relax, then expand under the sustained touch your hands offer. Your hands' input is just right to help calm the walls of the multitude of blood vessels protected under the ribs. Hopefully you'll feel when ribs start to expand. The response is usually very subtle. This is the perfect time to add in the stretch as you're lightly helping bread dough expand (though not really changing the dough's shape). Ribs often then begin to wiggle side to side and your baby will look like they are squirming. Follow your baby's lead; they will determine when they are done self-correcting their ribcage.

Collar bones and shoulders

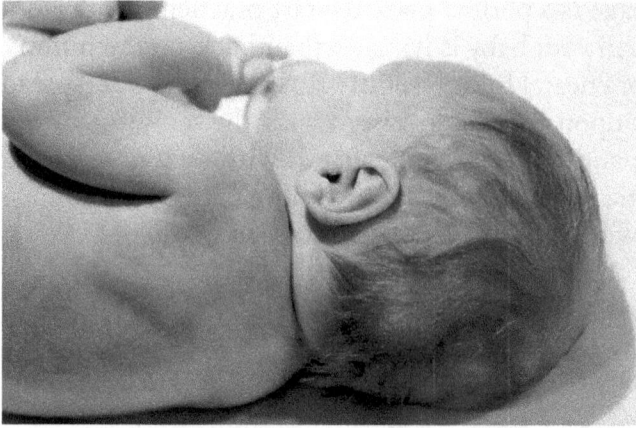

The neck can be stuck in a crunch from being positioned in the womb, but from absorbed forces from birthing. Your baby may or may not [fully] work these areas of tension out on their own. It's a false assumption that all babies do. Following is a road map to look, see, and help their neck, shoulders and upper ribs stretch and expand.

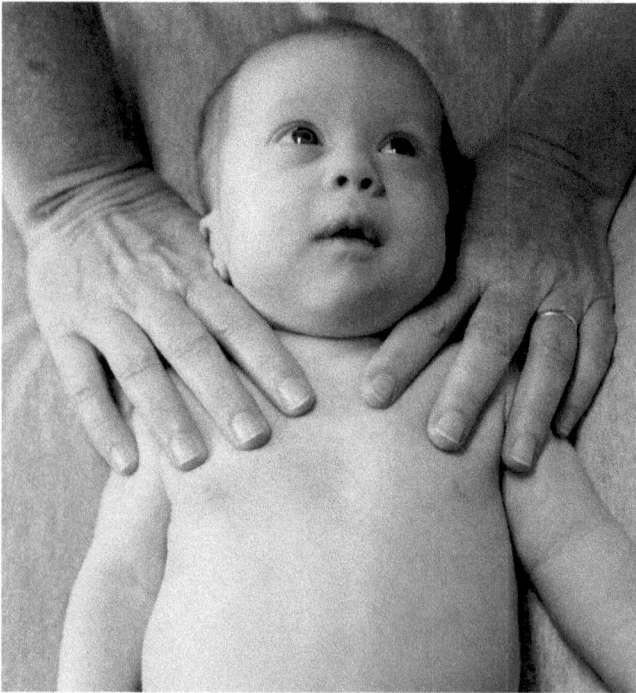

Continue to work on the rib cage from the top, including the shoulders and collar bones. Your first finger can feel for and then rest on both collar bones. With practice this can be easily felt just under the chin. This bone is attached from the breast bone to the shoulder. Many muscles attach to the collarbone, affecting the jaw, tongue, front of the neck, and even the core things that aid swallowing. It's essential that the upper ribs, shoulders, and neck expand from the forces of birthing.

Just as you did with the previous rib cage method, rest with this hand position and wait for their shoulders to relax, drop, and expand. Tissues of muscles, fascia, and blood vessels will respond when you give the *just right hold* enough time for your baby to self-correct into full rib expansion. This can be anywhere from one to ten minutes.

Side of Neck

The muscles on the side of the neck can be shortened and hold strains and muscle tensions still from the birthing process. Babies don't really have "short necks." Rather, they have compressed necks. The distance from the ears to the top of the shoulder reflects this reality. Compression is a result of the shock absorption into soft tissues of the body. This technique targets these side muscles specifically.

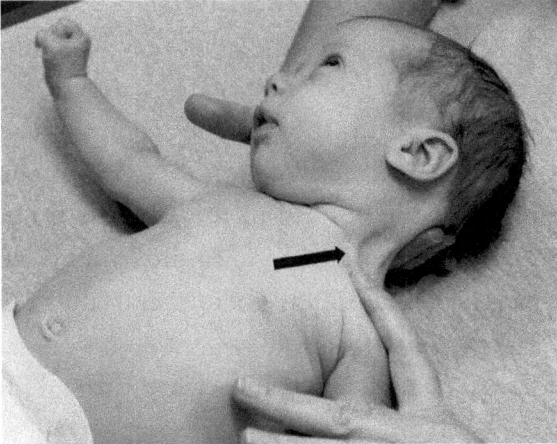
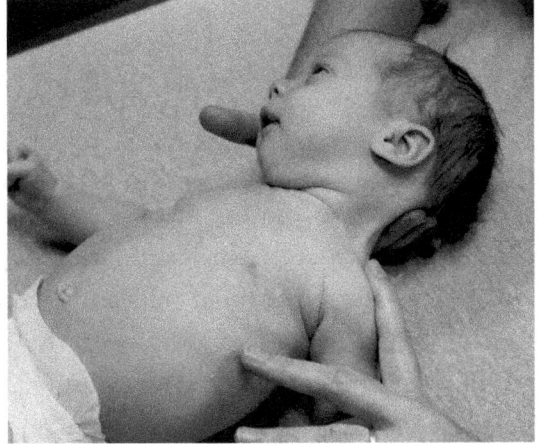

Before   After

Cradle your baby's head with one hand and use one or two gently placed fingers on the top of the shoulder. Apply the *just right hold* and wait for the muscles to communicate with your finger pads. Do not dig in or stretch the neck and shoulder. Instead, let sensory endings in your finger pads listen to the muscles' tension. Wait long enough with this hold and watch the shoulder drop as it elongates under its own power. You might notice some tension in the tendons of the muscles (see arrow in first photo). The second photo reflects the baby's self-correction and stretching her own neck under my waiting for the *just right hold* to take effect. This is the kind of stretch I prefer when treating torticollis.

This maneuver is very different then the traditional neck stretches we used to do when the mindset was the therapist was the "fixer" and the one responsible for correction.

DO NOT force such a stretch. This hold will help your baby drop their own shoulders. Baby should be calm, happy, and relaxed during this process.

Hyoid connections

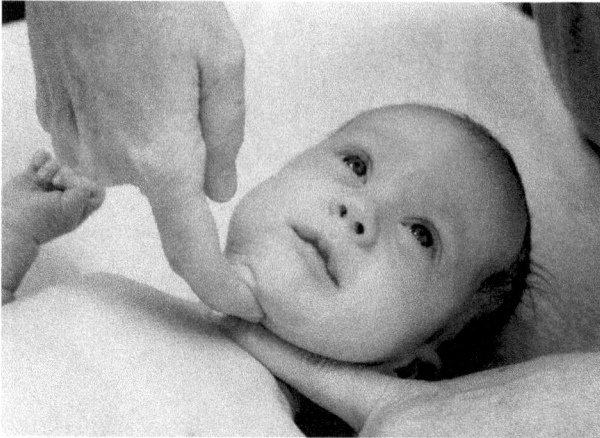

This stretch requires extremely delicate hands. Only try it if you are confident in your delicacy. The hyoid bone is a horseshoe-shaped bone on the front of the neck. This bone is still very immature and highly flexible cartilage on your baby. Still, it has the unique distinction of having over fifty structures attached. Four muscles on top of the hyoid form the tongue's floor. Other muscles project off this anchoring bone to the collar bone and breast bone, fanning out along the bottom of the jaw. The throat and inner ear structures have a relationship with everything attaching to the hyoid bone.

This stretch is most relevant when a tongue tie is present, before and after any surgical or laser release. Combining the *just right hold* with an uber-gentle stretch can mobilize and make pliable your baby's fascia tissues, which wrap and weave through all these muscles and soft bones.

To perform this stretch, make sure your baby is warm and well-fed. Being on their back securely on a table or your lap is the best place to try this. Lay one finger across the throat just under the chin and jaw. Remember, a lily pad on top of water is the amount of finger pressure to be mindful of. With the other index or middle finger or even your thumb, put the finger pad along the exact middle of the tongue floor. You'll feel this soft flesh from the tip of the jaw to the throat. Each finger remains in contact with the flesh and bone, and the tiniest stretch is applied, with the fingers moving away from each other. Your hands and fingers should look like the photo. Hold for 5-10 seconds. If you feel tight tissue resistance, you can repeat these one or two more times. Think of this as "yoga for your baby's chin, tongue, and jaw."

Please do not do this stretch if you feel uncomfortable or lack confidence. It is a simple maneuver to perform but requires very light hands and non-invasive touch. A gentle sustained stretch is the goal. You could ask a local bodyworker to work with you on this stretch to gain confidence.

Cradle Spine with Intention

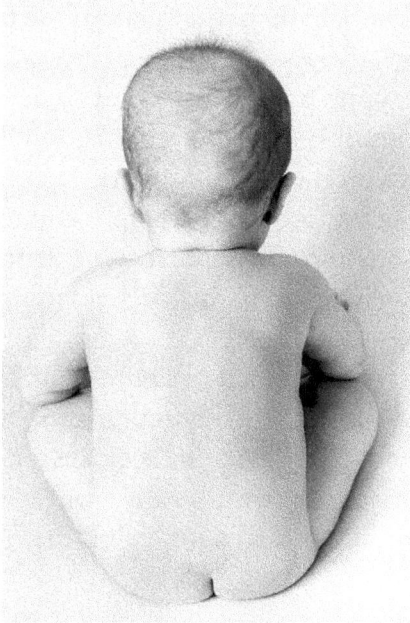

There are many bones that make up the spine, and even more connective and soft tissues. The body's core absorbs the shock of birthing or positional stress from being curled in the womb. Common sites of core compression are the bones between the hips (sacrum) and the base of the head. Tensions can also be stuck between the spine bones.

Your two hands can learn to feel tension down the body's core. This gentle hold and stretch allow all the spine's bone and surrounding connective tissues to decompress and unwind. A philosophy of gentle bodywork is to "follow the body and its tissues" as it relaxes and decompresses. This technique is no different. This method aligns with CranioSacral Therapy, proven to help even premature babies.

A common way to cradle a baby is to hold the head and bottom (buttocks). With a shift in your mindfulness of what your hands are doing, you can help them decompress core tensions. Hold your baby this way and focus on the sensations within both your hands. Tell your still hands to "tune in" with each other; one hand feels what the other hand feels. Feel the energetic connection traveling between your palms. **Do not bounce or jostle.**

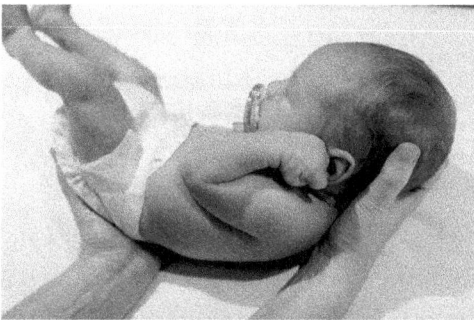

Using the *just right hold*, your hands provide the base and energy needed for this self-correction. One hand cradles the back of the head. The other hand fully cradles the whole bottom.

Imagine helping that bread dough rise by involving this unique approach. The mere "thought of lengthening" will help your baby respond to that intention in your hands. Refrain from applying a forceful stretch. Imagine a helium-filled balloon tied to a ribbon with a weight at the end, creating a line of stretch that stabilizes the balloon's position. Your hands holding the two ends of the spine provide a similar kind of sustained stretch. This hold aids in self-correcting connective tissue and muscle fibers in an unwinding. You should soon feel your baby's torso wiggle, stretch, and uncoil.

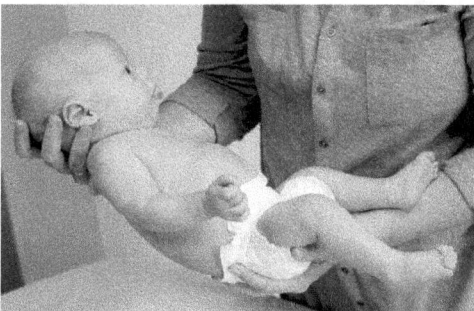

Backward stretch – often referred to as "Guppy pose"

Babies have several automatic reflexes that further help them move out of the fetal position. These movements elongate muscles and connective tissues out of tightly curled postures, lengthening organs and blood vessels. The "guppy pose" is a natural backward stretch of whole-body extension. This self-generated position helps them transition core tone from tight to loose and relaxed. It is a great way to promote tummy time, especially if your baby doesn't like being on their belly. This stretch is good to do before and after surgical releases of tongue ties, and it helps relax organs for better movement of food, waste, and gas bubbles. A baby can go into a guppy pose lying on their side, held upright, or when placed on a bed, floor, or table.

While the guppy pose is a natural and beneficial movement, it can pose challenges if certain structures in the body are too tight, impeding this whole-body action. One such structure is the deep-front-line fascia band, which extends from the middle of the tongue through the body's core and ends at the tailbone. Guppy pose stretches the front of the neck and throat and extends to the middle of the tongue, but it can be difficult if the front fascia band is not flexible.

Some methods of promoting guppy pose shared on social media should be left to the professional. Examples are:

- Holding a baby backward on an exercise ball.
- Holding a baby upside down.
- Any position where the head falls backward unsupported.

These listed ways tend to require skill and handling expertise. I have worked with many parents who "freaked" out over the thought of attempting these at home. These parents shared deep concern and fear of turning their newborn upside down or any way that appears they need to force the head and neck backward. These other methods hold the risk of being forceful and alarming. Plus, the head falling backward can reinforce the startle reflex. If parents feel uncomfortable placing their babies in such positions, they likely won't do them, regardless of professional recommendations.

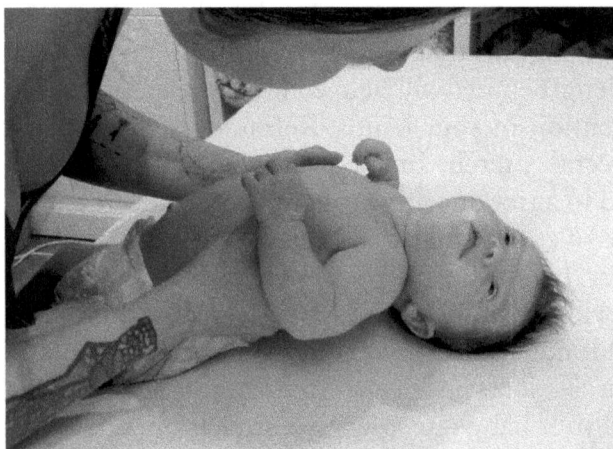

Teaching a mother to help her 8-week-old baby assume guppy pose

We found a better way. Our experience is that babies can get into a guppy pose if their body's fascia bands flexible and relaxed (either under their own stretches or through our assistance). When my fingertips form a soft bolster in the middle of the back, baby feels secure with their head and back supported by the table. Moving backwards is then under their active control.

Guppy pose – continued

The following sequence of photos shows the natural process of assisting this baby into backward extension by nothing more than optimal hand placement. You do not need to help them move backward or tilt their head. They will likely do it themselves.

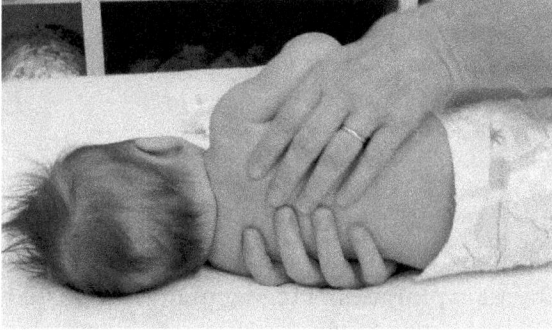

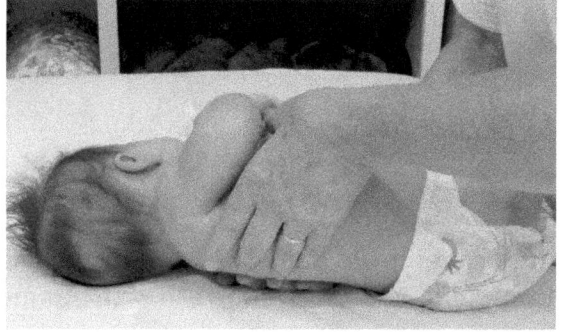

Begin by making a fulcrum with your fingers placed gently in the middle of the back, between shoulder blades. This triggers the extension reflex as you tenderly roll them onto their back.

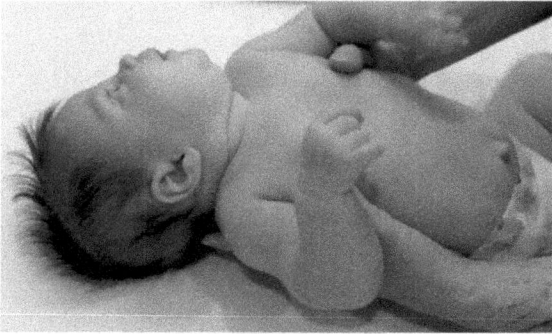

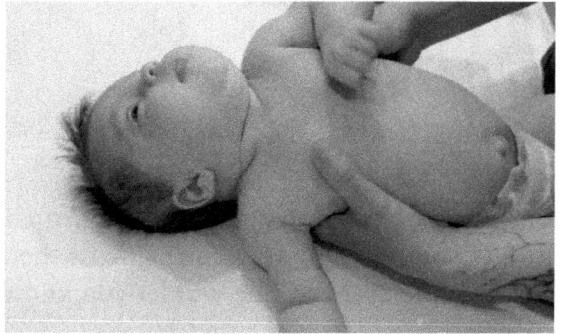

WAIT for their own system to recognize their body is ready to move backward. They may start by either arching straight back, or may turn their head to one side to start their motion. Keep your fingers softly placed in middle of back between shoulder blades.

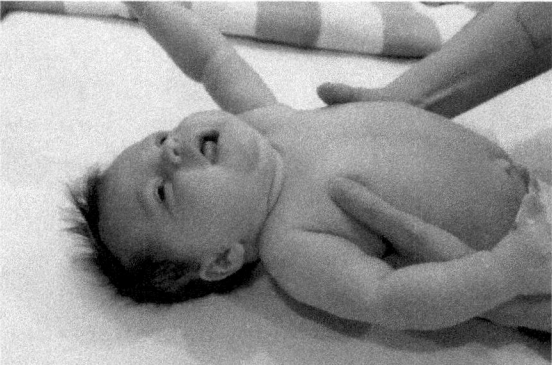

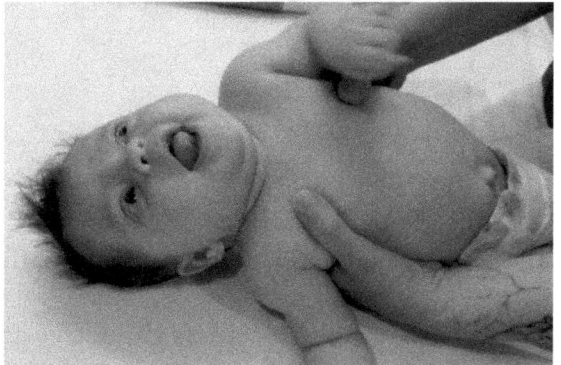

The pose can stimulate jaw and tongue movements.

Guppy pose – continued

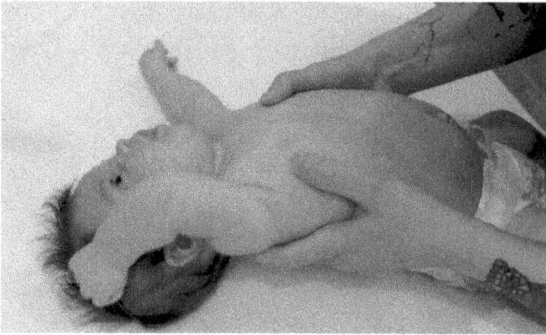

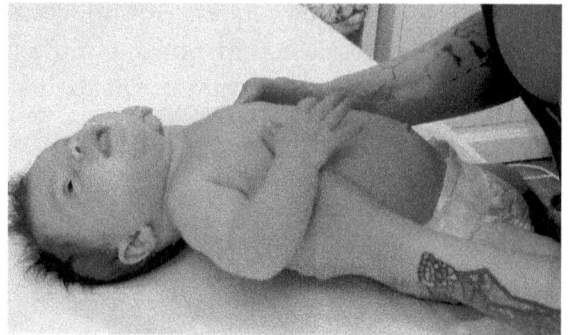

Your baby should not be stressed by this playful maneuver. Your hands form this fulcrum from cradling the ribs. Have fun with this movement exploration. Head remains supported.

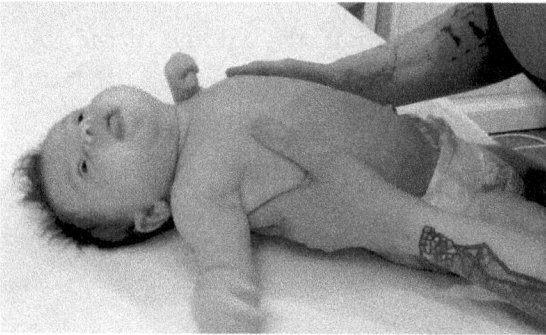

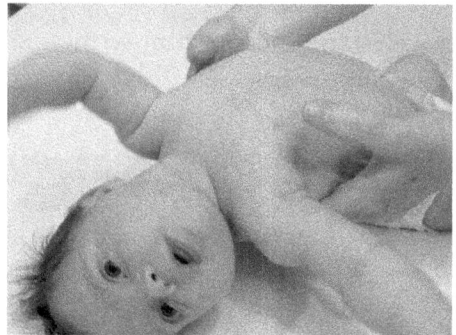

She may go back even further to "open" up her throat and neck, and then return back to the middle. She may go off to one side or the other. Continue to allow her own movements to guide the exercise. She will let you know when she's done.

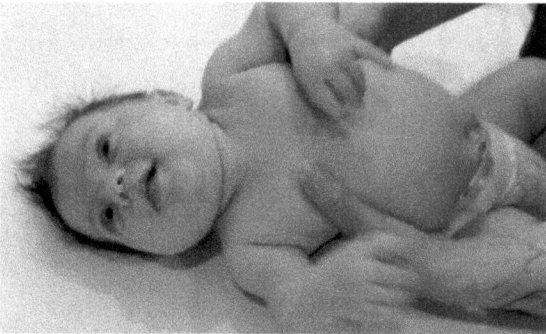

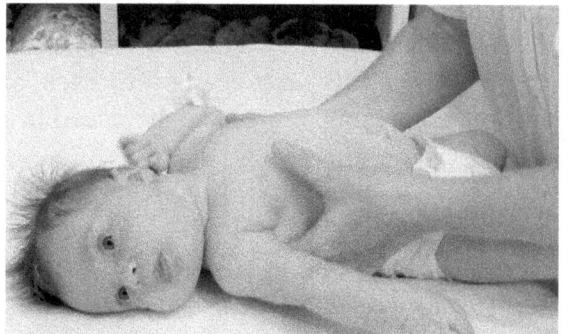

If her head turns either side, she's probably stretching of muscles on the sides of her neck. The longer you two play in this position, the more she works out herself.

This photo sequence depicts the active and dynamic play that guppy pose offers your baby. This pose should not be stressful… follow their lead.

Guppy pose – continued

- The key to helping your baby assume guppy pose is to cradle the chest. Your fingertips resting at the spine between the shoulder blades.
- WAIT to see if they like it and respond to being held this way.
- WAIT for them to sense their head on the table, then body gains a sense of security.
- WAIT for them to initiate the active moving backward into a healthy arch stretch.
- FOLLOW their lead and turn this time into playtime.

If your baby is consistently holding their body in an arch, it's crucial not to mistake that for a guppy pose. Babies typically move in and out of a guppy position until they achieve the necessary stretch. Then they should easily bring their body back to the middle and be balanced in their torso. However, if your baby seems 'stuck' in an arched backward position, it's a sign that a professional evaluation is necessary.

Don't do a guppy pose if the neck is still compressed into the shoulders. (Ears touching or almost touching shoulders). That means birth compression persists through the neck into the shoulders. Readiness for guppy pose is after ears and neck have moved away from shoulders, or after being assisted by a chiropractor or bodywork therapist with CranioSacral Therapy.

If your baby can't assume the guppy pose by themselves, it often means that [more] bodywork is needed to address fascia bands hindering their body movements.

If you have been successful with guppy pose, you can continue with whatever method you have found effective as long as your baby finds it fun and enjoyable.

Guppy pose should NOT distress anyone... baby or parent!!

Tummy
Digestive challenges: colic, constipation, reflux, ease of tract movements, grunting

Belly button and umbilical remnants

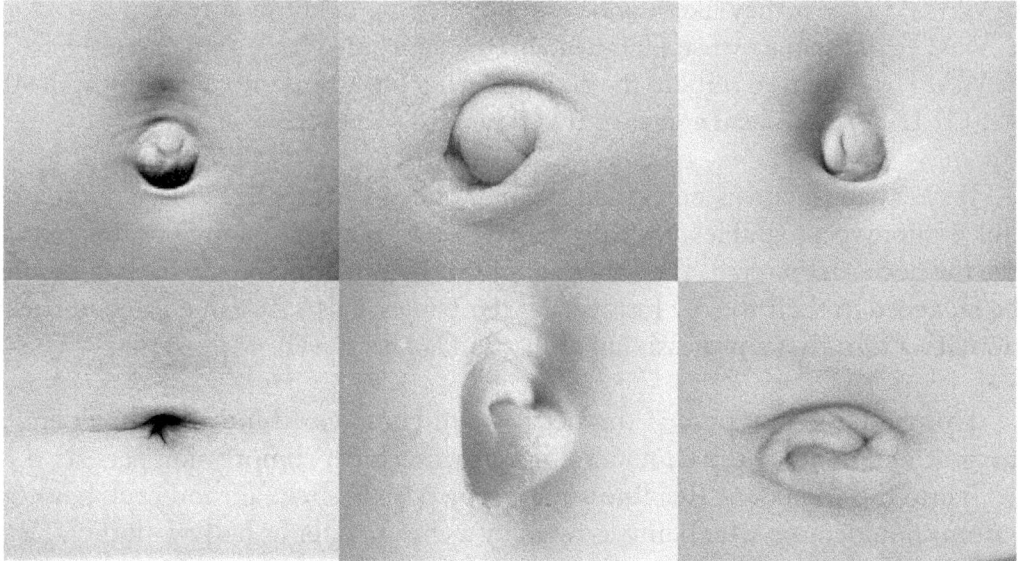

The belly button is the body's first scar, the retracted (drawn inward) end of the umbilical cord. Its shape is a direct extension of the fascia tissues that lead to and surround organs and blood vessels in the tummy. The left-over cord became a ligament suspending the liver to the tummy wall. Tension that persists in this and other nearby fascia tissue can be seen in the shape of the belly button. It can also be felt by your fingertips.

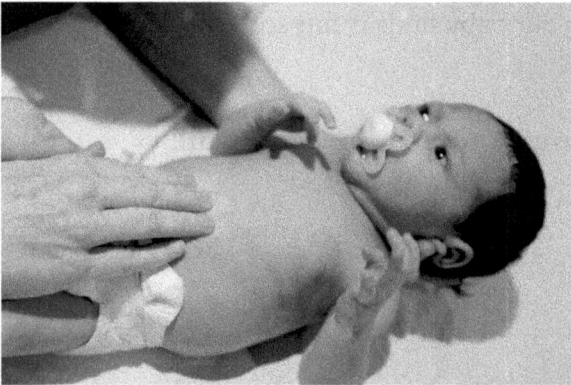

Stress and strain can happen with the umbilical cord during pregnancy by wrapping around limbs or the neck. A baby can grab and tug at it. In addition, when the cord is clamped while the blood vessels are still beating, much beneficial blood is left behind in the placenta. Complete transfer of placenta blood occurs before the cord stops pulsating has been proven. Research strongly supports the renewed practice of delayed cord clamping, though there is little science on the tension left behind in cord tissue. Bodywork wisdom is there can be tension behind the navel projecting up to the liver (where fetal blood originally traveled). Behaviors related to tense organs include colic, constipation, and self-regulation difficulties.

To help this area for your baby, gently place fingers over the belly button and let their tummy inform your finger pads of any pulls, tugs, or tensions that lie under the skin. Applying the *just right hold,* wait with your non-moving hand on spots of tension until these soften, relax, and expand, maybe five minutes or so. This technique also helps relax the liver, central nerves, and blood vessels. That's all that generally is needed. A bodyworker with expert training may sometimes apply more treatment here, such as visceral manipulation or myofascial release, if additional help is needed.

Deep Front Fascia Band

A recently discovered complex network of connective tissues (fascia bands) have been identified in the human body. These bands are considered the body's "soft skeleton" and work together to give the body its shape, strength, and stability. One in particular is a deep band in the front, a structure we now deal with for a tongue tie. Connecting the middle and floor of the tongue, fanning through the rib cage and chest, and traveling through the belly, this band comes to an end at the tailbone. Two branches then continue on down the legs to the big toes. The shape of the belly button and the tension of the deep-front-line can reflect distortions and tensions around the intestines, liver, stomach, and the clusters of nerves to these organs. Breastfeeding challenges, colic, and an intolerance for tummy time are common problems when this band is retracted and tense.

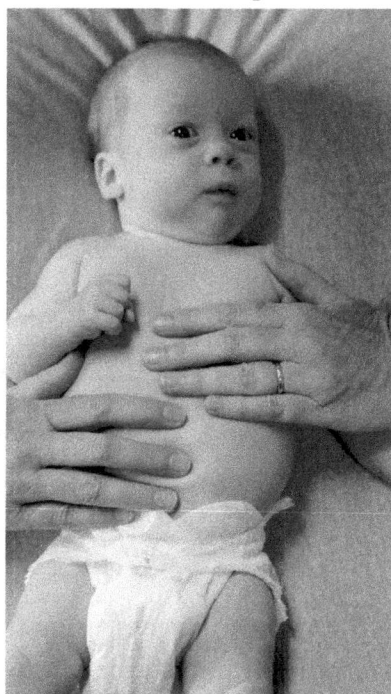

Lower portion   Upper portion

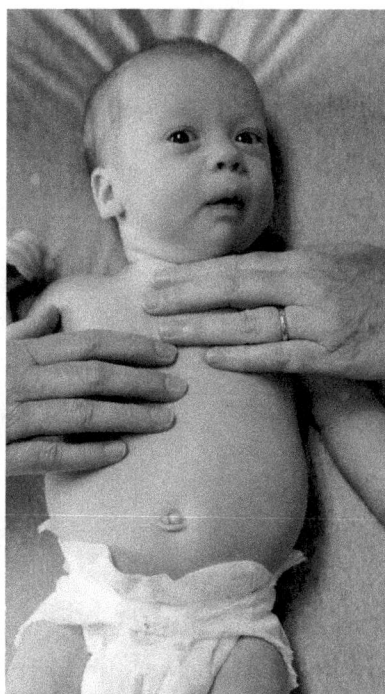

To work with this band, your baby only needs the *just right hold* mixed with a tiny stretch between your two hands. The goal is to gain some flexibility and slack in this band, not unlike stretching hamstrings on the back of our thighs. **But only a gentle sustained stretch is needed.** Here we treat the band in two parts, the lower and the upper. For the lower part, span your fingers from the top of the diaper to the bottom of the breast bone (sternum). For the upper part, span your fingers from under the middle of the jaw to the bottom of the breast bone and apply the *just right hold*. Appreciate any tension, and allow time for the *just right hold* to help your baby self-correct tissue expansion. If any stretch is needed, it will be tiny stretches between your fingers in small spaces. You should be able to feel more suppleness and pliability to that band after a few minutes of waiting.

Hand Placement for Intestines

When humans are stressed, blood vessels tighten. Babies are no exception, and in fact their immature system is even more prone to tightening. A significant amount of blood vessels are located woven between and behind the intestines. (About 25% of the whole circulatory system is here). Putting hands on this spot relaxes these vessels as well as the connective tissue surrounding the intestines. Turns out, this connective tissue is also what houses the "gut brain" mesh of nerves. Helping this complex region relax is one of the easiest and quickest ways to get into the "rest & digest" state.

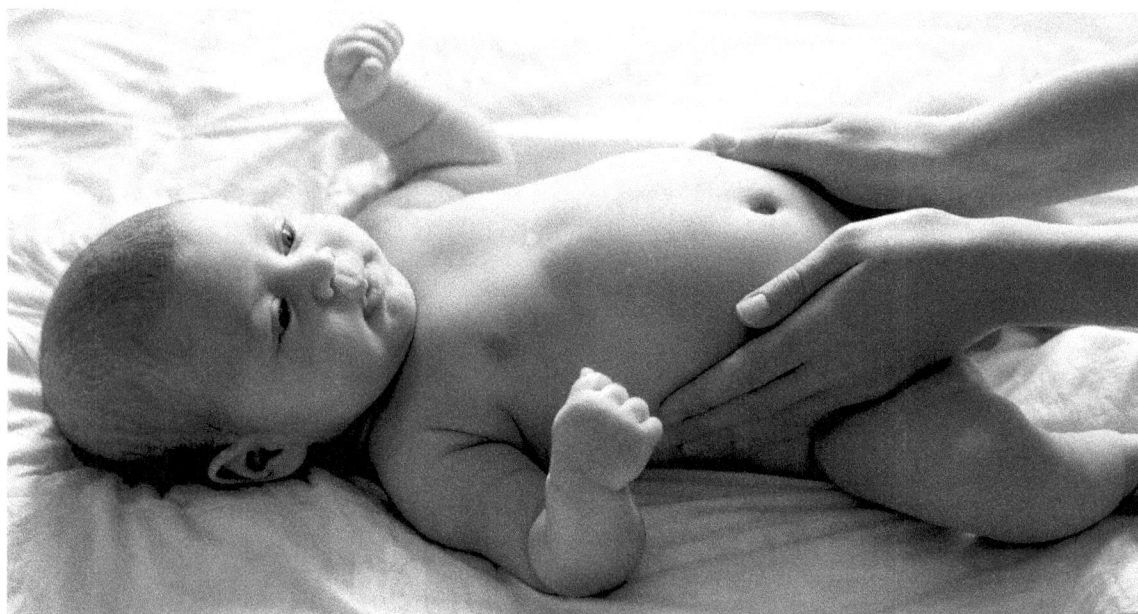

This technique puts warm hands covering the entire intestines, using the *just right hold*. Both hands cradle the lower tummy between belly button and the hips. Wait longer than you're used to waiting, which allows intestines and blood vessels together to soften, expand, and gain flexibility. Do not rub, massage, poke, or prod with your hands. Consider that span of your hands to be a wide acupressure point.

Holding this for five to 10 minutes will allow you adequate time to observe how your baby can self-regulate the tension in their intestines and the mass of blood vessels that weave through the length of the digestive tract. Holding this long enough can improve movement of fecal matter, ease the tensions related to colic, and even help them prepare to sleep.

Liver and Stomach

As with any mass area of blood vessels, organ walls can hold tension. When stressed (in an alarmed state), the organs feel tight. When not stressed (in rest and digest state), the organs are soft and flexible. Movement of food [milk] and waste happens best when organs are relaxed without added resistance down the digestive tract. The same effect of relaxing digestive organs (as we did with intestines) can be done over the liver and stomach. You can do both organs at the same time, or one at a time.

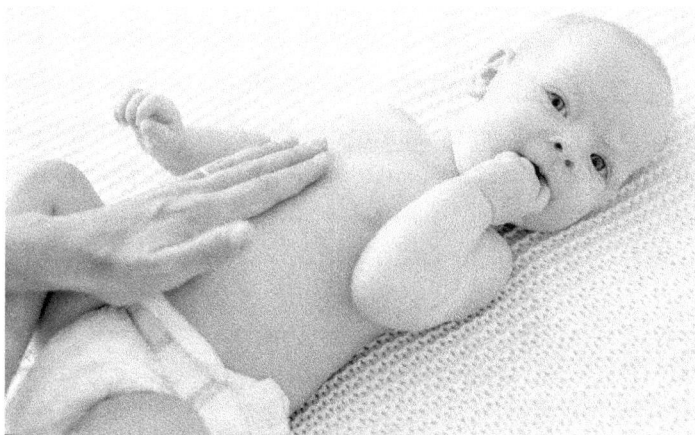

Liver

The liver is mostly on the right side and lies under the rib cage. Rest one hand on the front of the right-side ribs, covering all the lower ribs up to the nipple line. The heal of your hand covers the right half of the belly. The liver is a really big organ; the adult hand should cover most of it. Apply the *just right hold* and wait for a softening of the organ under your hand.

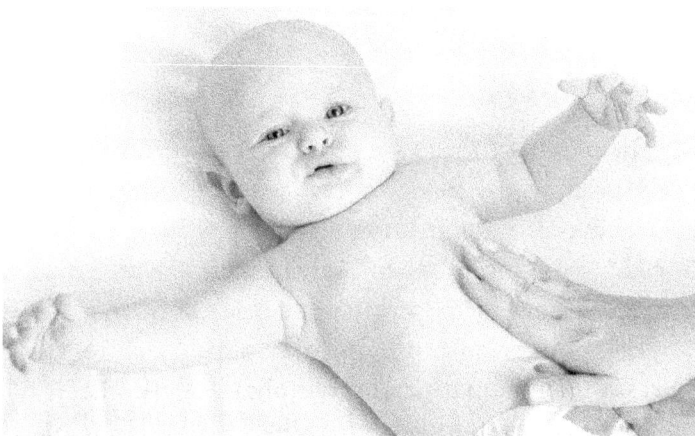

Stomach

The stomach is on the left side and is a smaller organ than the liver. Rest one hand on the lower half of the rib cage on the left side to locate the stomach. Using the *just right hold*, wait and follow the relaxation response as with the intestines. Apply the *just right hold* and wait for a softening of the organ under your hand.

Understanding and Helping Constipation

Parents understand instinctually the importance of their baby pooping regularly. If pooping doesn't come quickly or easily, a baby can be in a state of stress. This can be marked by fussiness, irritability, and grunting. The immature muscles in the intestines' walls need to develop mature contractions for regular bowel movement (BM) patterns. Becoming regular may take a few days, weeks, or even months. Babies can poop with every feeding or go once a day. The "normal" range of individual BM development ranges from several times daily to once every few days. As long as your baby is healthy and gaining weight, most healthcare professionals won't be concerned about fluctuating BMs during the first few months of life.

If your baby seems to be in pain or grunts or has to exert during a BM, it can reflect tension in the internal organs. They may express emotions, but they likely are not in pain as we adults know it. Passing soft poo can cause babies to strain, grunt, and cry. Not because they are constipated but more likely because of organ immaturity. True constipation is marked by hard, dry stool that is not easily passed. This tends to be more of a problem with formula than breast milk.

So, how can a parent know the difference between immaturity and actual constipation when the symptoms for both are somewhat identical? When to call the doctor:

- Obvious and repeated pain with bowel movements
- Passing ribbon or pencil thin stools; when waste is routinely hard and dry
- Blood in stool
- Lack of bowel movements accompanied by vomiting, fever, rash, lethargy
- Hard, distended belly

Routine advice has been given to parents to rub the stomach or provide a warm bath to stimulate the movement of bowel walls. Pushing legs gently into the belly and putting their legs through bicycle kicks has been known to help. However, when these massage tricks don't work, focusing on more specific areas has proven helpful. The following techniques are offered for parents to try to rule out if it's constipation or immaturity. These are conservative, non-invasive ways to help constipation before going to harsh medications and are based on sound osteopathic and lymphatic methods.

Bodywork for Babies techniques have repeatedly been proven to help breastfed and formula-fed babies trigger the movement of fecal matter through the intestines. Importantly, they bring relief from tight tummies and grunting without interfering with your baby's maturation process of the digestive organs. We encourage parents to allow some grunting and groaning from time to time.

The next few techniques are for when your baby is miserable and your gut instinct knows some natural relief would help.

Hip Flexors (psoas muscles)

The psoas muscle is a complex structure that connects the torso and the lower body. Tight psoas muscles are the primary muscle that bends the hips, and they also have fascia that support nearby organs. This is one of the main reasons babies' legs are held in the air when newborns lay on their backs.

The intestines are suspended partly by the connective tissues near these long muscles. If the hip muscles are tight, the tension frequently transfers to the walls of the intestines. This can add to the organ tension and increase the pressure the waste needs to move through the pipes. Helping these hip muscles (and nerves) relax has consistently reduced colic, constipation, and general fussiness.

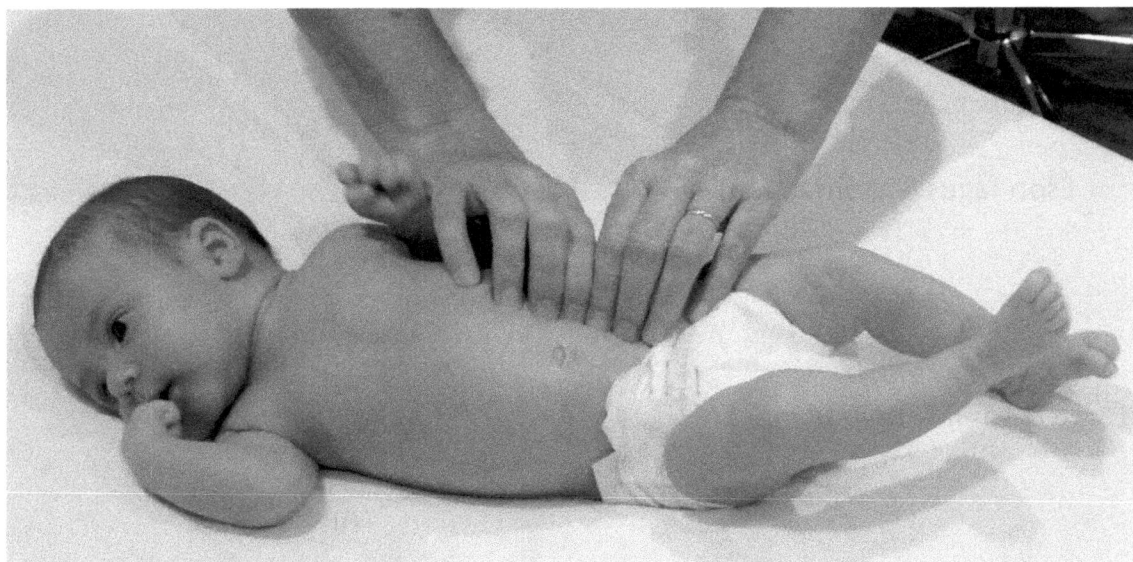

Gently place your fingers along the side of your baby's body, from the hip to the bottom ridge of the ribs. The flesh you feel is the belly of the muscle. Use the *just right hold* like you've placed your fingers on the top of a cold stick of butter. You are applying an acupressure hold here. Do not massage, prod, or jiggle your baby. Be patient and wait for the muscles, nerves, and connective tissue to self-correct through relaxation and softening. When this happens, the middle of the muscle will feel like soft, pliable dough. Legs will very often straighten and stretch, and the thighs roll outward. This area is very sensitive due to the mass of blood vessels and nerve branches woven through the intestines.

Response time can take anywhere from one to five minutes.

Digestive Sphincters

This map helps you locate the vicinity of each junction where parts of the digestive tract adjoin. Little muscles form rings or a drawing in of tissues that move in response to digestive signals. More specifically, these smooth muscles that alternate between constricting and relaxing are known as the digestive sphincters. Their job is to control the flow of fluids, food, and feces from one section to another.

Studying the digestive system and these sphincters can be a complicated endeavor. These next two pages are meant to simplify things for ease in understanding digestive and regulatory challenges your baby may face.

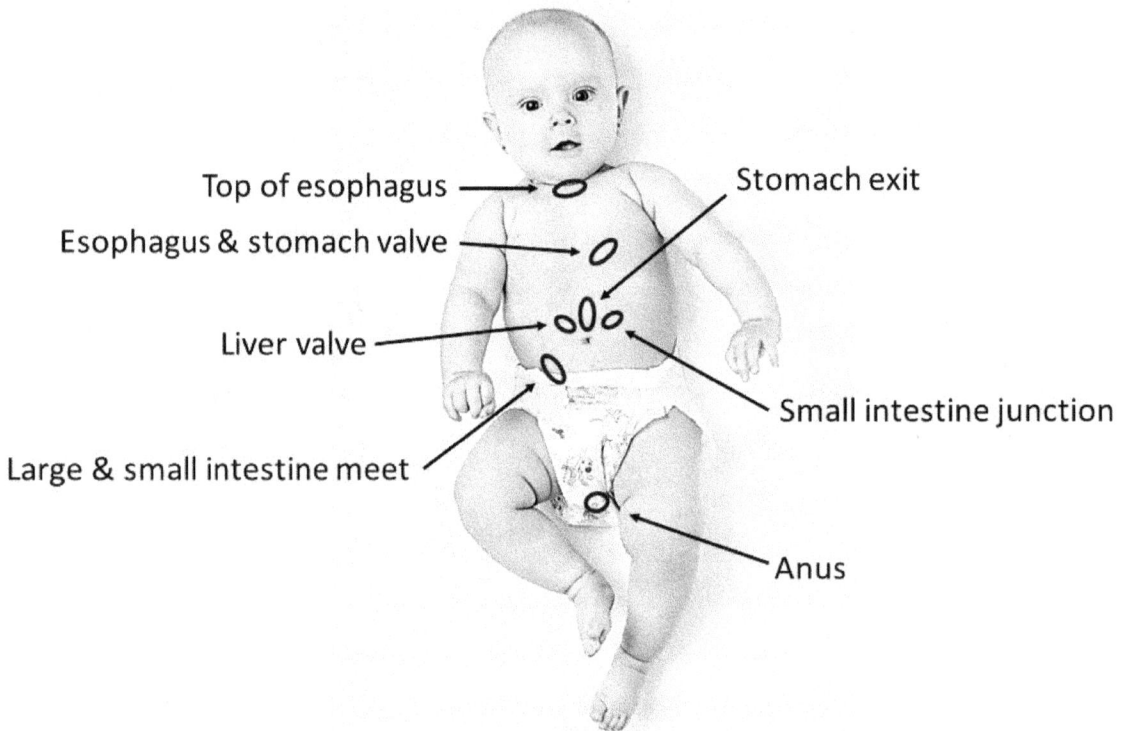

Locations of digestive sphincters

Colic, reflux, constipation, and general fussiness and irritability have all been consistently shown to respond to bodywork at sphincters. Helping sphincters relax and soften not only has been proven to help reduce these issues, it helps with overall self-regulation and even sensory modulation. Thus, bodywork at digestive sphincters helps the autonomic nervous system become more resilient.

A simplified version of treating each sphincter can be done in the following manner. Using the body map on p. 52, place a gentle finger in the vicinity of each sphincter. Acupressure and the *just right hold* is the only method needed. Rest finger pads lightly like a lily pad at any of the sphincter areas and patiently wait for a tissue response of self-correction and relaxation. Wait for the sensation of butter softening.

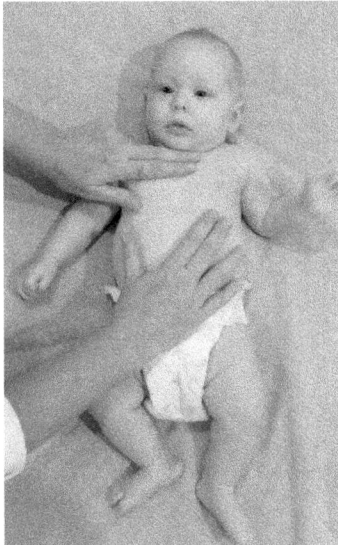

Throat under chin & top of stomach under curve of left ribs

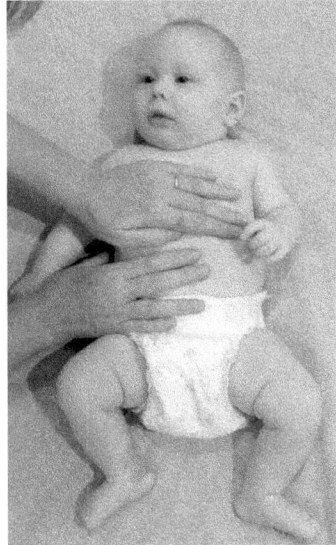

Top & bottom of stomach (~1" above belly button)

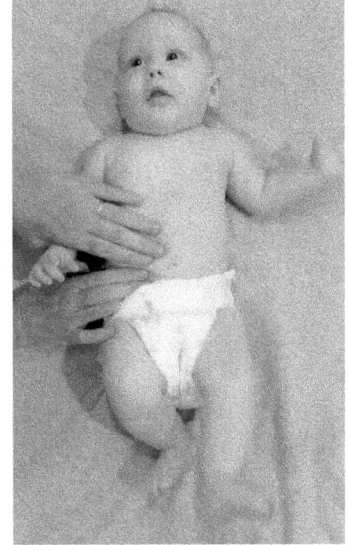

Liver valve & small intestine junction are left & right ~1" from bottom of the stomach

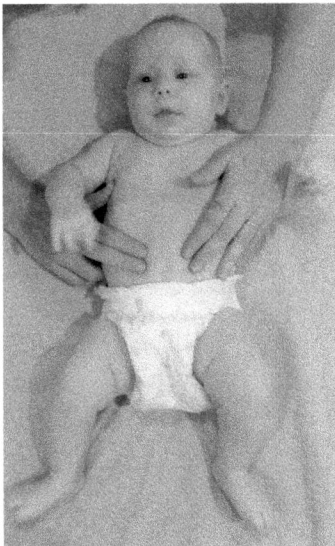

Liver valve & small intestine junction

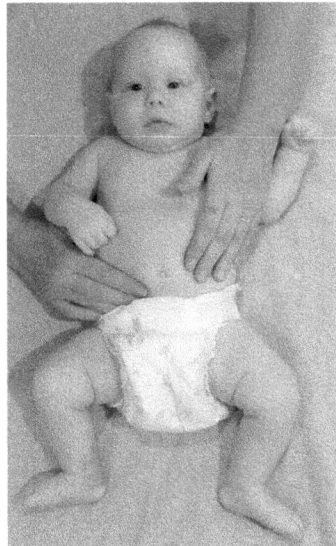

Small intestine junction and ileocecal valve

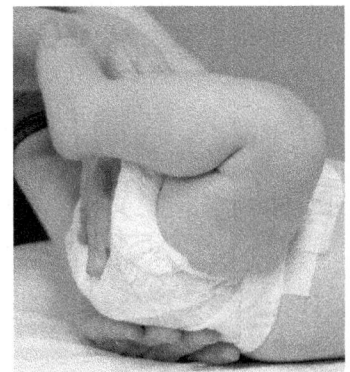

Anus: can apply through diaper or with a gloved hand

Two sphincters are treated simultaneously in each photo to show efficiency in treatment, but you can treat one at a time. Getting to know if any particular sphincter area holds tension regularly can communicate the reasons for reflux, colic, and constipation.

Evacuate the Bowels

Part I: Feel for Fullness

Locate the start of large intestine: half-way mark between belly button and right hip bone. It is the **X**

With gentle fingers, feel fullness along Length 1; feel from **X** upward toward the right-side nipple.

Stop under dome of ribs (black curved line), bringing your fingers to Corner 2.

Turn Corner 2 and gently feel fullness along Length 3. This length of large intestines is about a finger's width above the belly button.

Feel fullness to Corner 4, just under the rib dome & in line with nipple.

Turn corner and gently feel for fullness moving down toward hip along length 5.

Keep your fingers at middle of Length 5; begin Part II

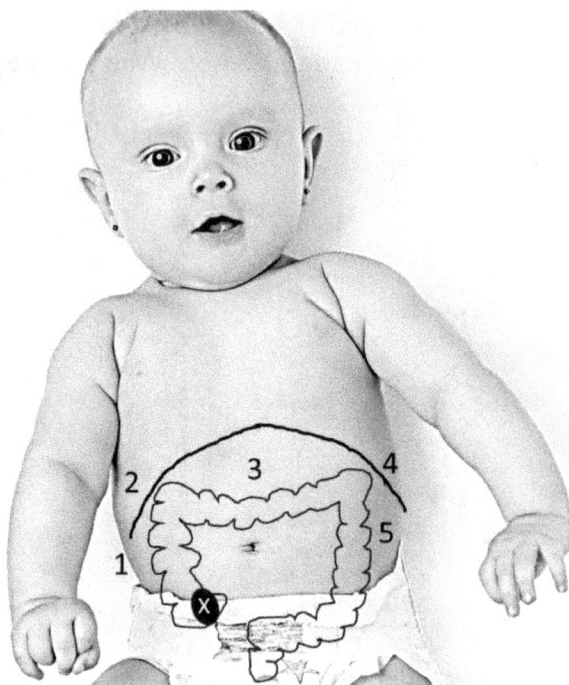

Part II: Evacuate Poop

Once the fullness of the large intestine is appreciated, you will gently "milk" fecal contents towards the rectum (below 5), which curves off of the large intestines. Move in reverse order of Part I.

Begin with your fingers milking down Length 5 towards the left hip.

Once back at Corner 4, rest fingers at this corner for a bit, helping any fullness turn the corner. The corners are often where the most tension is found.

Move slowly backwards along Length 3 milking contents towards Corner 4. Slowly move from Corner 4 to Corner 2, milking contents towards the left from the right side.

Once back at Corner 2, rest fingers a bit, helping any fullness turn this corner towards Length 3.

Moving down Length 1, milk contents upward towards Corner 2, evacuating entire Length 1 back to **X**

Your touch should only be as gentle as lily pads on water to help intestines relax

Limbs and Special Spots

Armpits Depths (upper ribs)

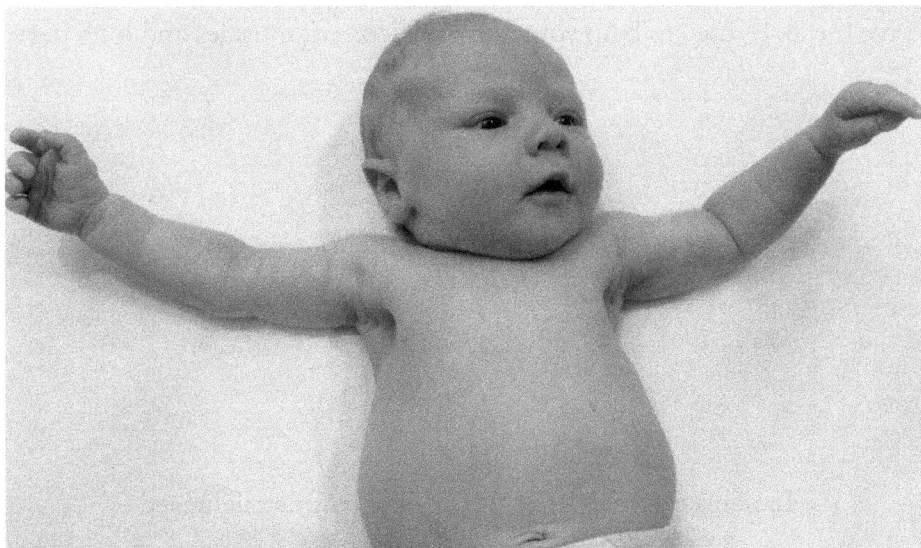

Internal tension of the lungs and a tight rib cage can be indicated by "deep" armpits. The inward pulls often come from upper rib muscles that are still retracted from birth or fascia band tightness. While much of the armpit can be relaxed with the rib cage treatment method already reviewed (See p. 36-37), a gentle whole-arm release can be a beneficial addition.

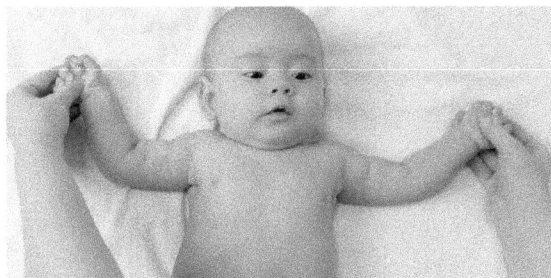

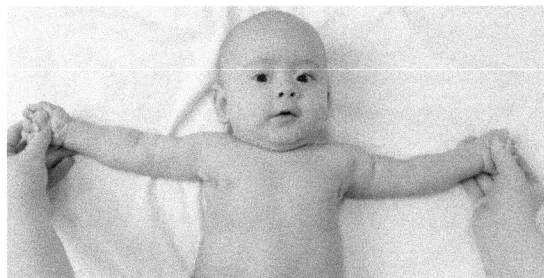

Arms

Hold one or both arms at the wrists or fists, and apply the *just right hold* with a very gentle stretch away from the body. Wait for your baby›s arms to soften and relax under their own power, under the sustained stretch. Do not force or overpower your baby›s arms. Take your time and allow your baby's arms to lengthen in their own time and control.

You can take before and after photos to appreciate any change to the depth of the armpits. Any change reflects the expansion of the rib cage and shoulder, and the tissues and organs underneath. Your baby will decide if they want arms to go straight out to the sides or up overhead. Allow time for your baby's movement decisions to lead the exercise.

Legs

Tight hips from being curled so long in the fetal position can keep the legs tense and the pelvic muscles shortened. A general stretch to the legs in the same manner as the arms can give the assistance to help your baby self-correct muscles and long nerves off the spine.

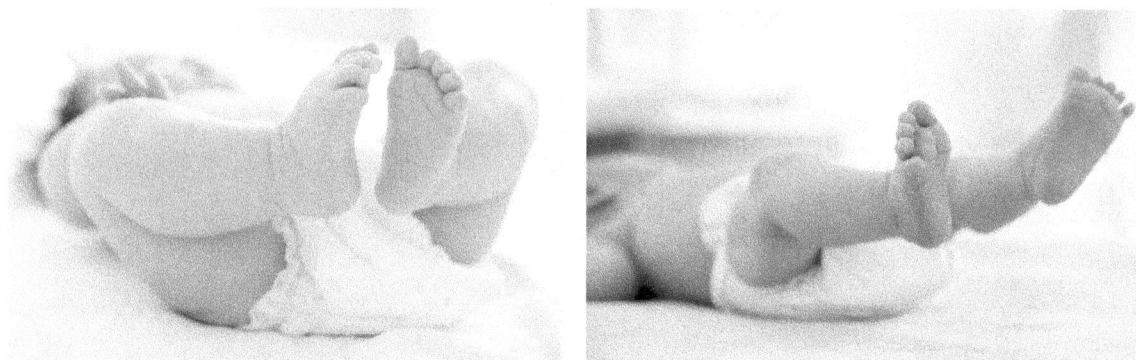

Tensions can keep legs stiffly bent or stiffly straightened.

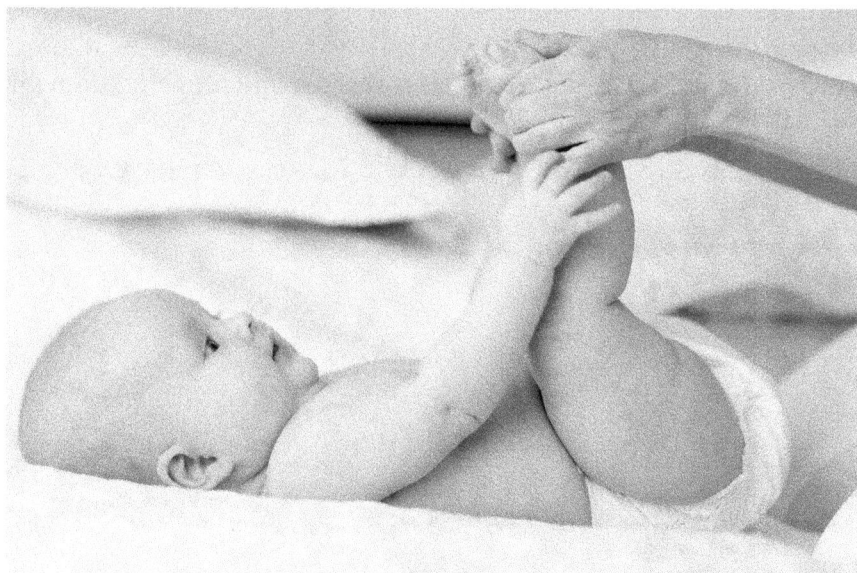

Gently hold one or both feet and ankles and apply the *just right hold* with a very gentle stretch away from the body. Hips can be bent or straight. Follow your baby's lead. Wait for your baby's legs and knees to soften and relax under their own power, under the sustained stretch. Do not force or overpower your baby's legs. Take your time.

Hands – Feet – Ears

Tight fists, curled toes, and stiff ears can reflect tension in the body's core or organs. Clenched fists can indicate hunger or be a reflexive reaction to sensations. The intensity and duration of tension demonstrate the degree of internal stress. Persistent tautness in these end parts may be due to nerve strains in the neck, shoulders, and rib cage. Tension through the legs and feet can reflect similar strains through the long nerves off lower spinal cord or organs. Stiffness of the ear cartilage can be translated from the nerves in the head and body organs. You can use simple acupressure tips at hands, feet, and ears to help your baby's inner world relax.

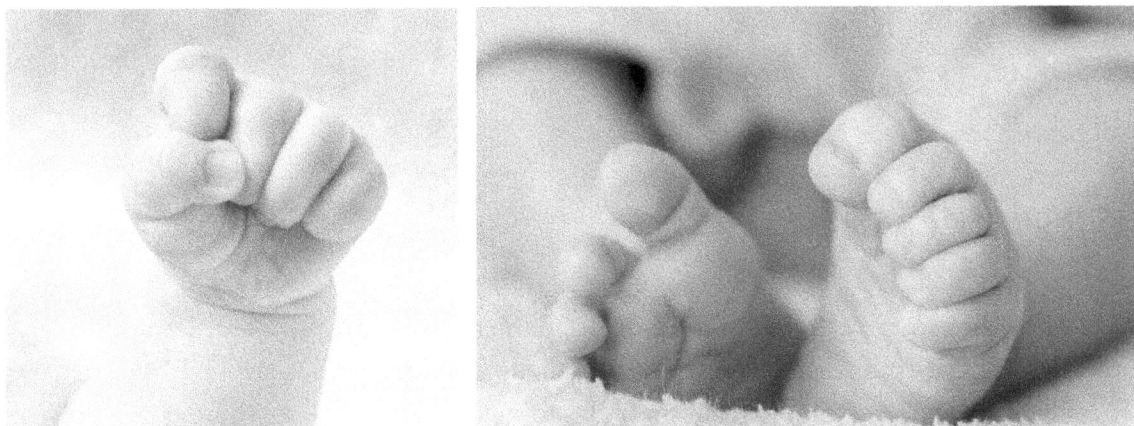

Acupressure to limb parts

Acupressure, a wonderfully uncomplicated technique, is a staple in *Bodywork for Babies*. This can be seamlessly integrated into your caregiving routine. To apply, simply use your thumb and finger to create a gentle 'pinch' like the *just right hold*. Instead of using both hands to hold a limb area, you're now honing in on a smaller and focal tension spot with a thumb or a thumb-finger pair. Maintain a light touch pressure, allowing enough time for the stick-of-butter melting sensation. Remember, the softening occurs due to your assistance dilating blood vessels, which relaxes muscles and connective tissues.

Gentle, sustained pressure is key. Less pressure is more effective. Too much pinch or pressure will actually cause blood vessels to tighten in protection. It's crucial to understand that rubbing or massaging is not advised. Moving hands can also actually increase tension. So if you try massaging and your baby is not calming, the rubbing is having the opposite effect of what is intended. Instead, the goal is to apply steady pressure on the spot and wait for tissues to self-relax. When babies are stressed, usually less sensory input is better.

Keep in mind, you're not responsible for the relaxation. Your baby's tissues and organs will relax on their own in this way if you create the just right input. Trust me and try it.

Specific reflex points on the hands and feet match particular organs, bones, and body systems. However, we will not worry about what spot corresponds to what organ. That's a job only for academics. Knowing the complicated reflexology maps or corresponding nerve endings in the soles of the feet and other appendages is not needed to offer help to your baby. Instead, simply feel for the firm points and apply acupressure. The goal is to help that spot soften and relax.

Thumb Webspace

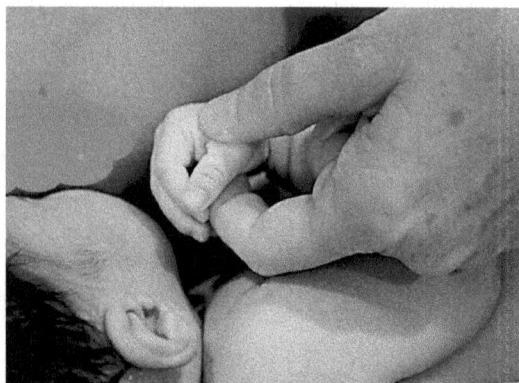

One particular spot we frequently treat in our clinic is the thumb side of the hand. The chief relaxation nerve (vagal nerve) branches to rest within the muscles in the thumb's website. A gentle acupressure in the muscle belly can activate a whole-body response of relaxation by stimulating this pressure point.

Soles of Feet

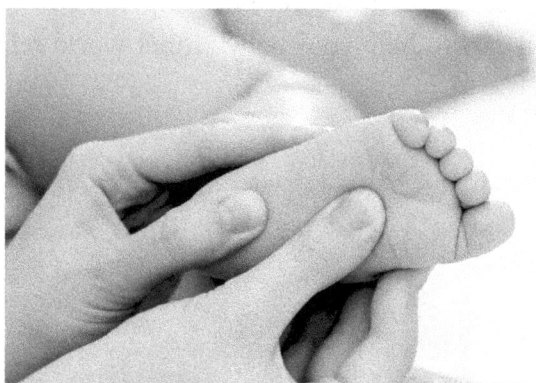

Babies' soft and immature muscles and ligaments in the feet are highly responsive to acupressure. The technique of applying gentle pressure and the just right hold can effectively relieve tension. Instead of massaging the feet, simply touch them with the intention of locating areas of increased tension (firmness). Apply gentle pressure and the just right hold, and wait for the tension to resolve. You will be working with tiny body parts, but it's reassuring to know that acupressure is a safe and beneficial method for your baby's relaxation.

Do not rub or massage. Instead, learn to find the tense area and hold this spot with a pressure that feels like waiting for the butter to melt, a gentle and gradual sensation. If you press too hard or rapidly, you risk increasing the tension. The muscles, hands, and whole body can relax given enough time holding the acupressure. Learn to feel the difference and you're all set.

Ear Acupressure and Ear Stretches

Babies' ears are incredibly soft and pliable because history of stressors is not yet reflected in tough cartilage (as felt in adult ears). Compare your ear cartilage to your baby's and feel what life does to our ears. Cartilage toughens with age, and there's nothing we can do about that—or so we thought. Even older ears can regain softer flexibility through acupressure at firm cartilage spots.

It is amazing to learn that so many nerve endings in the ears correspond to many body organs and long nerve meridians. (Nerve meridians are like a highway map system of the associated wiring through the body.) Acupressure calms nerves, relaxing the blood vessels, organs, and muscles served by these nerves.

Place pads of your thumbs deep into the ear valley, touching the opening of the ear canal. Apply the *just right hold* combined with a soft acupressure pinch. Your pressure

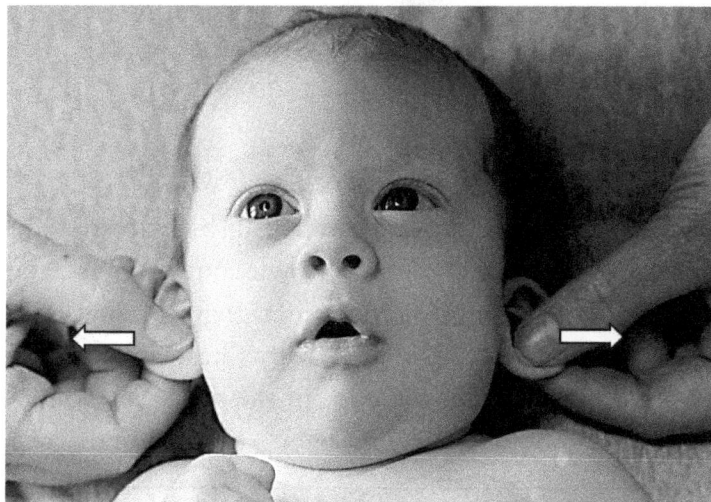

should match the tissue's resistance; not too hard of a pinch to cause discomfort. Do not distort the shape of the ear. Wait for the response of the ears to becoming soft and pliable. After that initial softening, apply an extremely gentle pull straight away from the head. (See arrows). Hold for five to ten seconds.

Should your baby become distressed by this, assume your pressure or pull is too much. Back off and adjust your touch and pressure. Softly pinch like holding a stick of butter and wait for the melting feeling. That is the value of combining CranioSacral with acupressure methods.

This ear technique has a proven track record of helping to relieve pressure in the ears, particularly in situations like airplane travel. It can also stimulate sinus and eustachian tube drainage, providing additional benefits for your little one's comfort.

Head / Neck

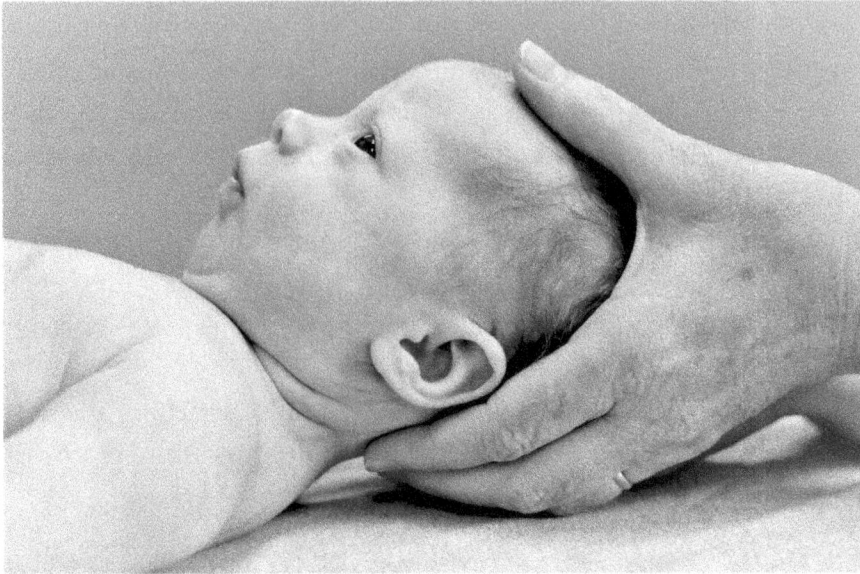

Head Self-Decompression From Neck

This classic bodywork technique empowers your baby to stretch their head, neck, and shoulders out of core tightness. Under their own control, your baby will be the one doing any active movement. The most important thing to know is the placement of your index finger pads. Cradle the back of your baby's head with your fingertips resting where the head and neck meet at the lower edge of the head. You will apply only the *just right hold*, which provides a good base for your baby to complete this self-correction.

Do nothing else but hold this position. <u>You will NOT be stretching the neck!</u>

Patiently wait while supporting the head, using the *just right hold,* and watch how your baby can decompress their head from the shoulders. You might see the neck get longer (spine decompression) or the head start turning side to side. This hold can even help your baby go into a nice guppy pose (full backward stretch). Allow your baby to control all those movements. You can't hurt your baby when you simply hold the head still. Patiently wait long enough to activate stretching under your baby's own power.

Be mindful that your hands only hold the head so the neck can move. **<u>You are not the one who will lengthen the neck</u>**. Nothing else needs to be done. The best results occur when you hold this position for a sustained time (1 to 5 minutes) and patiently wait for your baby to work off the still, stable base provided by your hands.

Cranium Reshaping

Babies can develop flat areas on their heads if they are placed in the same position for long periods. The pressure from the surface that makes contact reshapes the soft skull bones and the connective tissues. Premature babies are prone to flattening, especially on both sides, since their thinner bones and connective tissues can grow into the shape of the pressure point. Multiple birth babies (twins, triplets, or more) have an increased risk of head misshaping. The newborn's neck is too weak to move the head off those spots. Other factors can contribute to flattened heads, such as too much time spent in baby swings, bouncer seats, or car seats. However, time spent on the tummy during waking hours is a highly effective and recommended way to help heads remold by minimizing the pressure on one side of the head.

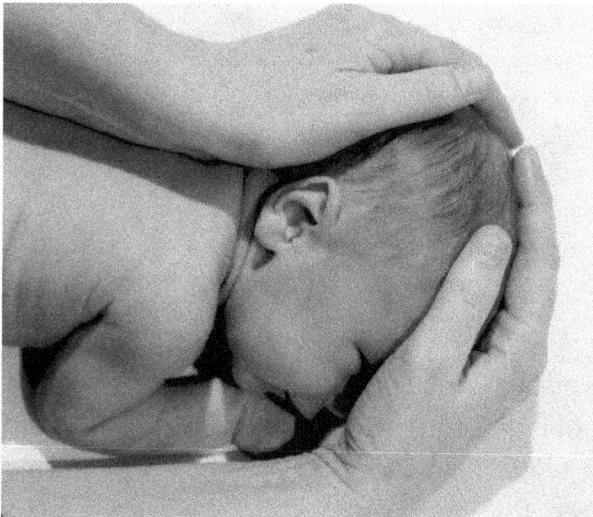

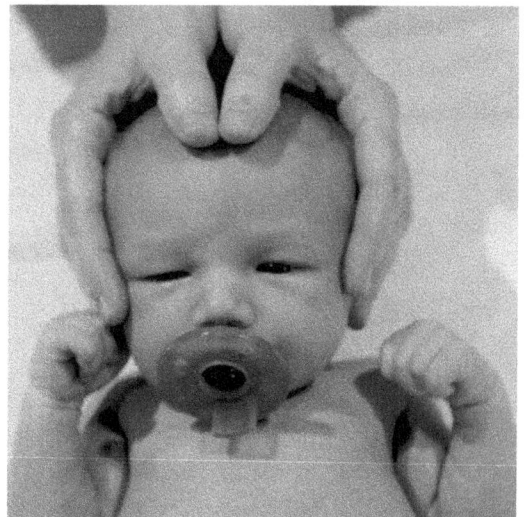

This osteopathic/CranioSacral technique uses the *just right hold* to help the head self-correct from typical molding from birthing. The fascia hold the shape of the head since those tiny bones are only floating and growing within the layers of tissues. Embracing the head in this manner intends to assist the natural dynamic expansion of connective tissue layers under and around bones. You don't need effort or force, only the gentle *just right hold*. The caring warmth you convey in your hands is enough to assist blood vessels and fluids to expand, aiding in the remolding process.

Cradling the head with your hands. The key is to start by feeling the shape of the head and understanding that its tissues are dynamic. Your baby's brain is rapidly growing under soft bones, which are still floating within the fascia container surrounding it. As you hold the head, become aware of the tensions within the skin and tissues underneath the scalp. Similar to how you held the head and buttocks to assist the spine in unwinding, your therapeutic hold on the head can help tissues release the compressive energy that may have caused any flattening.

Torticollis (head tilted or turned to one side) and prematurity (which lends to weaker neck muscles), are two common contributing factors to flat spots. Pediatric therapists who practice bodywork methods regularly treat these conditions, often in conjunction with head molding techniques.

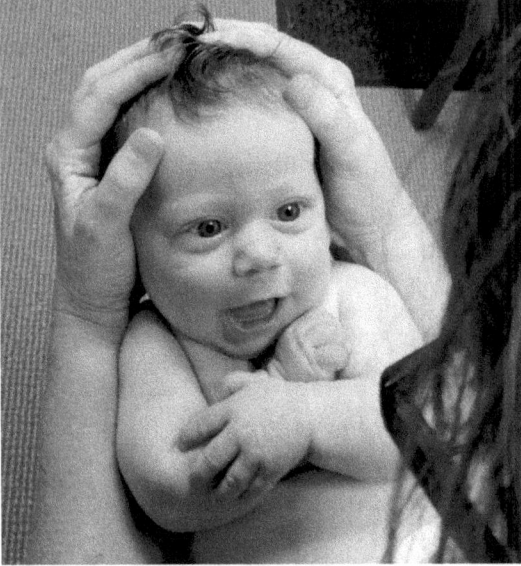

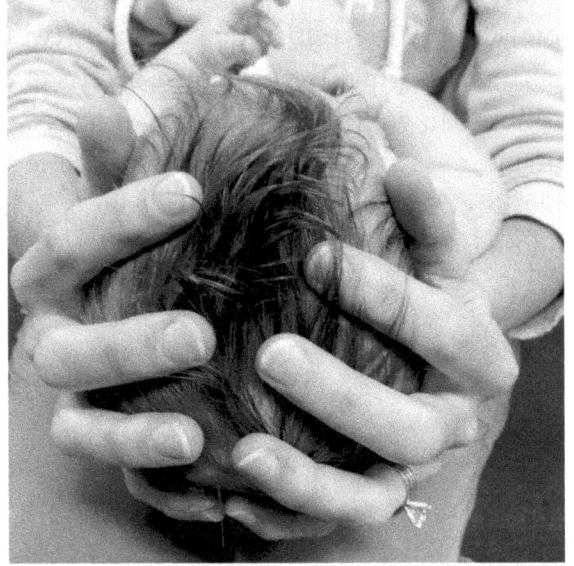

If your baby's head shape requires more extensive molding correction, it's advisable to seek the expertise of a CranioSacral therapist or cranial osteopath. These professionals, with their experience in gentle head remolding, *can provide effective* solutions. But if you're not able to immediately access professional help, the time you spend holding your baby's head can be beneficial and prepare them for future bodywork sessions. Remember, the sooner bodywork can be given to your baby's misshapen head, the faster and more lasting the results. Your proactive approach as a parent can make a significant difference in your baby's head shape.

A Word About Head Reshaping Helmets

Foam-filled helmets (cranial orthosis) are used to gently [re]mold a misshapen head, correcting the shape of the skull during a phase of rapid growth. The best age for a helmet to have the best effect is between 4 and 6 months of age, though success has been reported as old as 14 months. Helmets may be best used when the head shape is moderately or severely altered. Mild misshaping has been shown to resolve with mindful repositioning, manual therapies, or a combination of both.

It's important to note that helmets only correct the skull bones, not the additional bones that extend beyond the skull›s tissues that form the face. This means that certain aspects, such as ear placement, eye shape, and jaw placement, may not be fully addressed by helmet wearing alone. Similarly, helmets may not generally correct bone overrides, which are felt as ridges where two bones meet. Helmets also don't correct body fascia pulls that influence head and neck shape.

Bodywork for Babies, which includes CranioSacral Therapy, osteopathic manipulations, and similar methods, is an alternative treatment option that addresses the head in its entirety. This can be particularly beneficial if a helmet fails to achieve the desired end result in head remolding.

Parents deserve the information to make the best choices for their family's situation.

Ways to Help Your Baby's Head Reshape
(see also p. 71–76 for positioning for holding and playing)

- Prevent a flat spot from developing by changing the position your baby rests their head throughout the day. Be mindful of the head's placement when laying until they have complete control of their necks. (About four months).
- Body wearing, side-lying, and a variety of holding positions reduces pressure on the head.
- During sleep time, alternate the sides which their head is placed night to night. Or place your baby down with the head towards the top of the crib one night and the foot of the crib the next night. Babies tend to turn their head to things that interest the eyes, often the doorway where you'll walk in and the light coming into the room.
- Once they can turn their head, you can coax them to roll off any flat spot by grabbing their attention to their opposite side with a fun thing to look at.
- Limit the amount of time your baby is placed in sling seats or bouncy chairs, especially during the first three months of life. These "containers" have been shown to place adverse pressure on the heads of young babies.
- Have your baby spend time on their belly, either placed on your chest as a newborn, or fully on the floor after the fourth trimester. Keep in mind that your baby's neck is commonly too weak to master tummy time until after the third month. Never force positioning on the floor. If your baby becomes stressed and does not tolerate being on their tummy at all indicates that bodywork could be beneficial.
- Use of pillows or rolls around the head or face or neck is not recommended during sleeping. However, head and neck supports are perfect to support baby's head while in a car seat until the neck is strong enough to keep the head at midline. Don't let the head fall to either side for long periods of time in a car seat.

Head Shape Variations

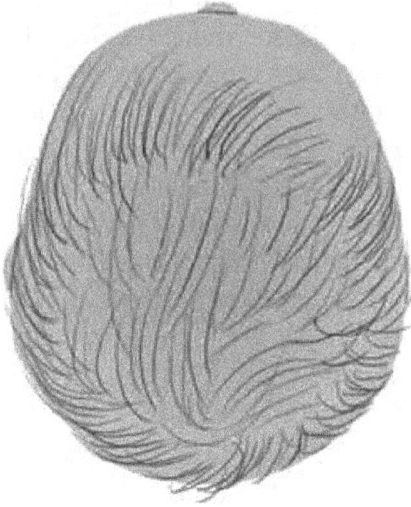

Typical rounded shape

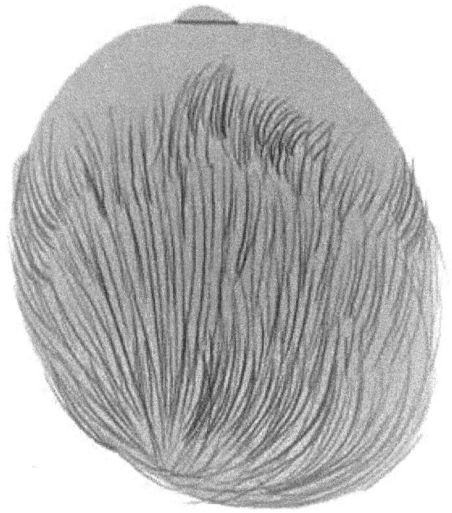

Flattening emerging on side

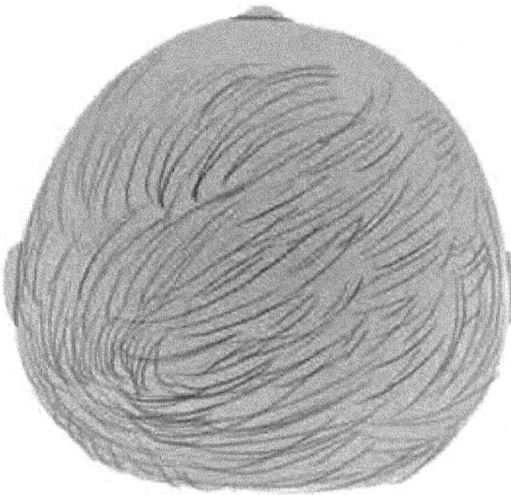

Flattening emerging on back

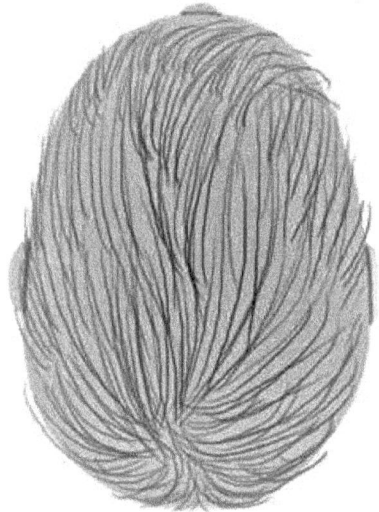

Flattening occurring on both sides

Track Progress of Head Reshaping

Weekly photographs can track your baby's head shape recovery from birthing and positioning. Compare changes in symmetry with grid lines superimposed over photos you take of your baby from these perspectives. (See p. 23)

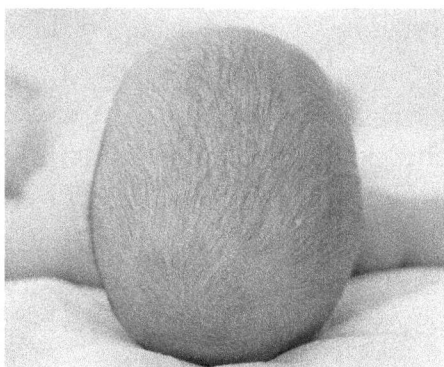

This view highlights the shape of the top of the head. Try to photograph the circumference of the crown as well as the placement of the ears. (Keep your fingers off the top of the head when you capture this photo). Using grid lines superimposed, track ear position and shape of the crown's four quadrants.

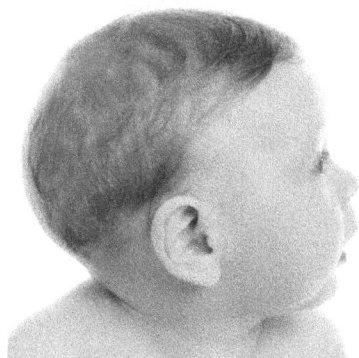

This viewpoint highlights the shape of the forehead and the curve on the back of the head. Often if the back is flattened, the forehead is protruding. Compare the profile shaping with tracings on paper placed over the photo and draw an outline of the shape of the head and face.

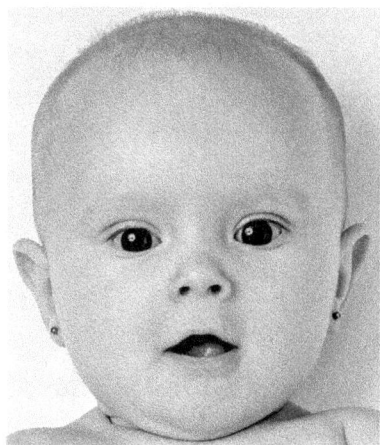

This viewpoint highlights the bones that shape the face, form the eyes, and reflects the tissues that suspend the ears. We are naturally drawn to the symmetry of parts. Use the grid lines from p. 23 and superimpose these lines to compare symmetry of the corner of the eyes, tops of ears, cheek bones, and corners of the mouth.

Face and Mouth

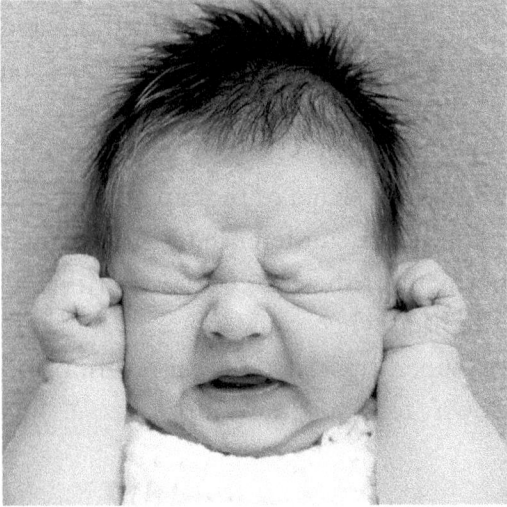

The face and jaw can also be compressed, most commonly from a combination of birthing strains into immature jaw muscles that can't yet overcome the forces. This contributes to babies' inability to open their mouths wide enough for a broad and deep latch. When the jaw is tense, it can cause painful clenching and inefficient munching at the nipple during breastfeeding. When a mom has to help the mouth open wide enough to cover the nipple, the jaw's mobility needs attention.

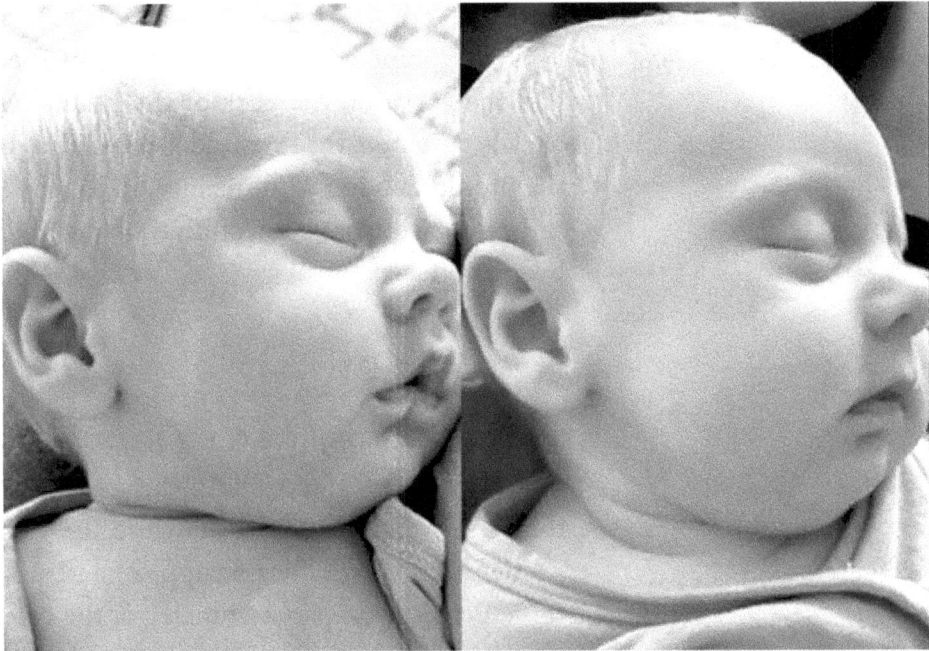

Before   **After**

Here are Before and After photos of a baby with a significantly compressed jaw. The lower lip pulled inward can reflect the jaw's compression and tension. The second photo is after a single treatment of bodywork. I have taught many parents how to stretch the jaw for such a correction. And yes, this baby slept through his treatment!

Decompress the Jaw

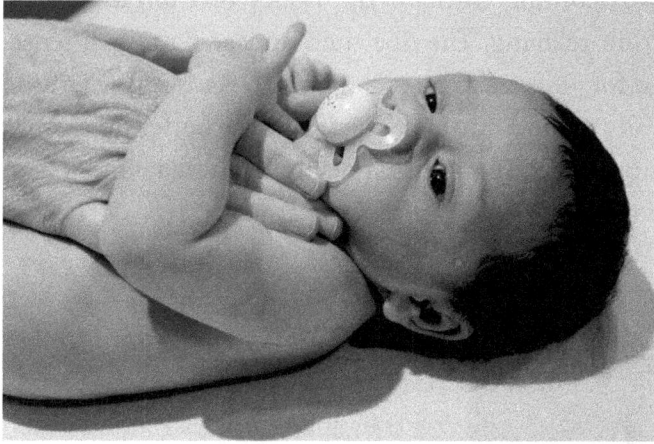

When you have to open your baby's mouth with your fingers for a wide enough latch, try decompressing the jaw instead. Opt for a gentle stretch to the tissues that move the jaw. The key is to be precise with your finger placement on the jaw bone and be extremely gentle with a stretch. This promotes jaw relaxation and helps reduce tension in the face muscles.

Locate the edge of the jaw and place 1-2 fingers pads in the middle of each side of this small bone. Keep in constant contact with the bone and gently stretch downward towards the feet. The key is to hold a minimal stretch, and NOT use a significant force. (A big force will cause the jaw to pull back even more for protection.) The *just right hold*, where you find the perfect balance with any tissue resistance, allows the blood vessels in the muscles to expand and relax under their own power. When the release happens, it will feel like a subtle stretch to taffy. Match the resistance the muscle gives you.

Relax jaw muscle

Gentle acupressure into muscles that open the mouth (if it is tight) can further help relax the jaw for a wider mouth opening. Place a finger pad (middle finger) on the

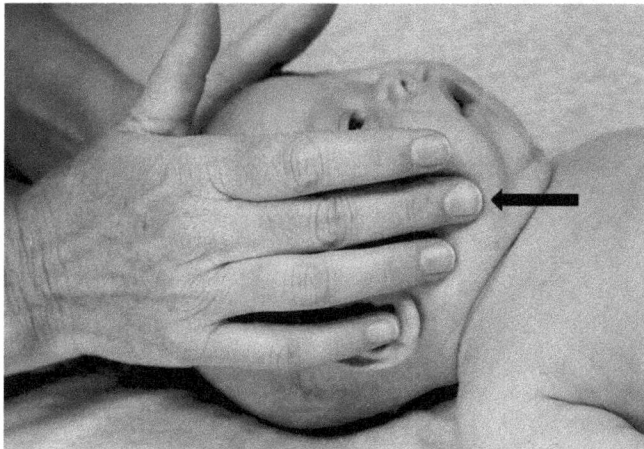

belly of the muscle in the middle of the cheek. (arrow) Appreciate the presence of any tension. With lily-pad-on-water gentleness, apply the *just right hold* and acupressure. This can take several minutes to complete itself. Wait for a softening response from the muscle(s) and the cheek to relax. Do not massage.

Relax Upper and Lower Lips

Compressed or retracted nerves coming through the bones of the face to the upper and lower lips can block lips from relaxing. The lips then appear flattened, tense, and tight, hindering the best lip flange for a deep latch on the nipple. Acupressure to the upper and lower lip can help relax the nerves and muscles. The result is a better lip closure and seal around the bottle or breast nipple, creating optimal negative pressure and a base of stability for the tongue to work from.

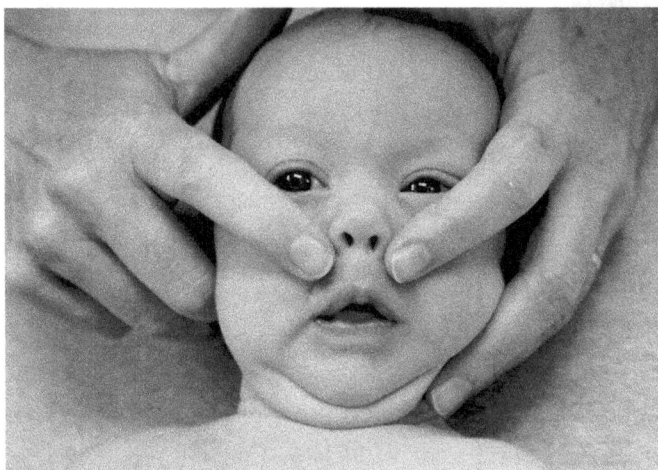

For the upper lip, place finger pads to fit the width of each side of the upper lip, just under each nostril. Apply the *just right hold* and acupressure. Wait for the softening and relaxing sensation of the mouth and middle face.

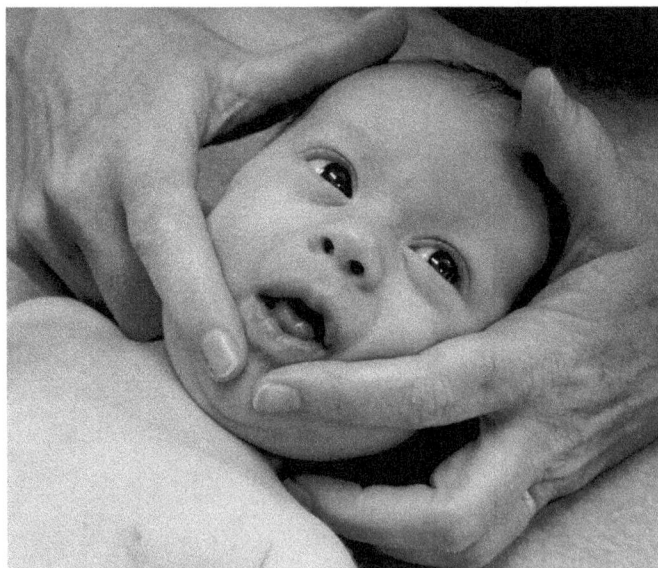

When it comes to the lower lip, place the length of both index fingers along the curve and in the middle of the jaw. Your fingertips should be close to touching, but not quite. Apply the *just right hold* and wait for the lower face and skin over the jaw to soften and relax.

Hard Palate of Mouth

The roof of the mouth (hard palate) is an area your baby needs and likes pressure. Usually, their own tongue achieves this with rigorous sucking and elevating to press into the palate. If a tongue tie is present or the suck is weak, enough pressure may not be exerted upward. A "bubble palate" can result from a significant tongue tie. The bubble is a deep curve in indentation to the hard palate. In addition, the soft palate is muscle and connective tissue that extends backward off the hard palate into the back of the oral cavity, forming the ceiling of the throat. During swallowing, the tongue pushes against the soft palate, and the muscles tense to push food backward and down to the esophagus. The soft palate then elevates to close the nasal cavity, preventing food from passing into the airway.

The hard palate comprises two paired bones that meet at midline to form the skeleton of the face, creating an arch. Like all other bones of the head and face, the hard palate is influenced by the tension of the surrounding fascia and the connections with adjacent bones. Mechanical compression, especially when the birth is a "face presentation" or the baby's crown is off-center of the cervix, can create imbalanced tensions in the fascia and bones of the entire oral cavity, including the palate.

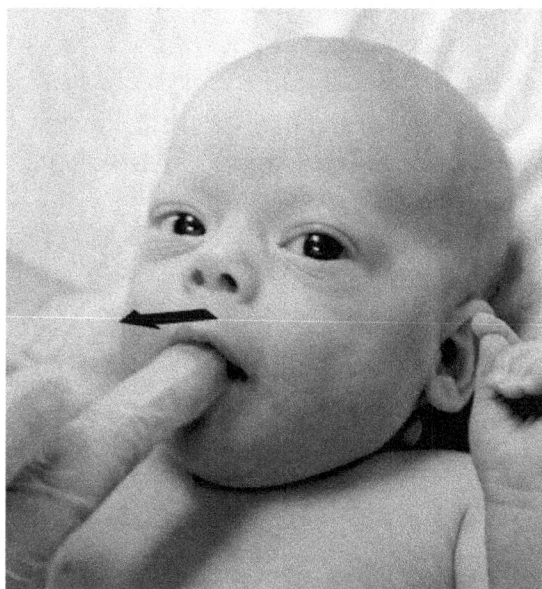

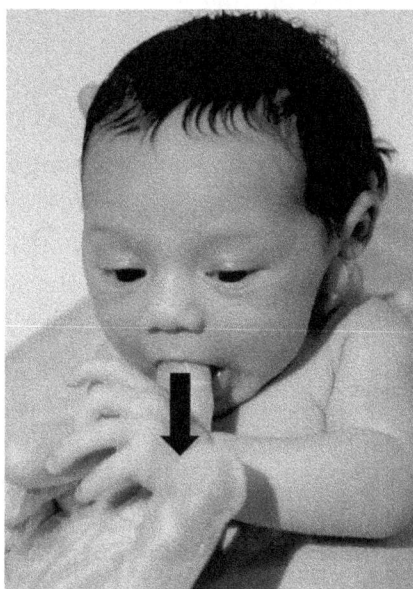

Gently rest your index finger on the front end of the hard palate, just behind the gum line. (You may use a glove if you feel the need). Apply the just right hold with your finger pad resting in the middle of the roof of the mouth. Do not put your finger further than halfway to avoid setting off any gag reaction. A gentle stretch between the hard and soft palate can actually reduce a hyper-gag reaction, and help guide the tongue to a stronger push upward. This method decompresses the hard palate from the soft palate. Only a thought of stretching will give the "perfect amount" necessary for tissue mobilization. No need to overpower bone or tissues here. Hold and wait for tissues to soften under their own power.

Suck training

Treatment involving suck training and swallowing liquid and food should involve a licensed professional qualified in oral therapies. Practice scopes that allow these professionals to work with dysphagia (swallow dysfunction) have traditionally belonged to speech and language pathology. Occupational and physical therapists and rehabilitation nurses can also hold specialized training in oral feeding therapies. The risks of aspiration, disorganizing the autonomic nervous system, or creating an adverse effect upon maternal bonding are too great for the untrained practitioner to casually engage in feeding training, suck training, and intra-oral work.

However, bodywork can help the movement components of tongue, lip, and jaw action (on relaxed neck and shoulders) in non-nutritive sucking. Non-nutritive suck uses the same movements as nutritive sucking. CranioSacral therapists typically have adequate training in mouth work methods to be of valuable help in this area.

Furthermore, the mouth is a sacred space for every single person. It holds and possesses many fundamental qualities of being human. Breathing, eating, speech, and communication, as well as a guardian for emotions, make the mouth a door to one's soul. Because of this, anyone trying to help a baby's mouth must recognize how sacred trust is placed in our hands assisting their oral health and wellbeing.

When approaching your baby's mouth, their hands guide entry. Lay a finger on the lips and allow mouth to open. Wait for your baby's tongue to meet it, allowing them total control of the finger's entry beyond the gum line. Once the finger is accepted and engaged by the tongue, let them show you their pattern and coordination. The ideal suck pattern includes: curling the tongue sides with a furrow in the middle, a strong pull, backwards, pressure into the roof, tight closure of lips, and a rhythmic cadence. When you baby is less than four months old, they show the strength of suck through a reflexive sucking. Meaning, when something is placed on their tongue, they automatically begin a suck pattern. Later, they begin to have full control over what their mouth does and choose to suck or not.

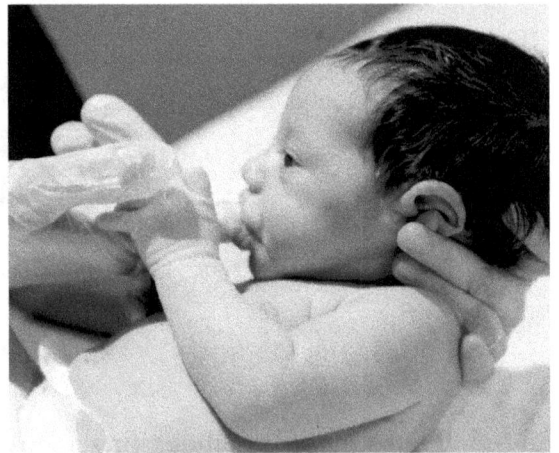

You can help your baby strengthen their feeding suck by exercising their non-feeding suck, without the stress of managing fluids besides saliva. Suck training helps strengthen. I like working on this in sloth position. (p. 72)

Positions for Holding and Playing

Holding and playing with your baby can naturally offer sound bodywork effects. Until your baby is moving their head, neck, and body independently, being mindful of several things can help set a healthy start in body resiliency. What your baby lies on, how long they lie there, and what effect their position has on muscles, organs, and sensations will become more into your awareness. The following holding and playing positions are included here to guide you and everyone caring for your baby.

Helpful Hold for Burping

Your baby teaches you the best way they like to be burped. If burps come hard or delayed, it could mean that the walls of organs or the sphincters along the digestive tract have added resistance from surrounding tissues. The sphincter at the top of the stomach releases the air, but hopefully not the contents. Spit-up is often milk still in the esophagus and has not yet entered the stomach. Reflux is when stomach contents are regurgitated. Both issues can be eased by helping the fascia around sphincters free from tension and strain between organs.

Recognizing the signs of trapped air bubbles is essential. These signs include crying, clenching fists, drawing legs into the belly, or arching back. When you notice these signs, it's a cue to help these tissues soften and relax, which in turn helps the digestive system reach the "rest and digest" state. This allows air and fluids to pass with better ease.

This hold helps gently compress the rest and digest nerve (the vagal nerve) as it travels from the base of the head along the neck and behind the jaw. This way of burping

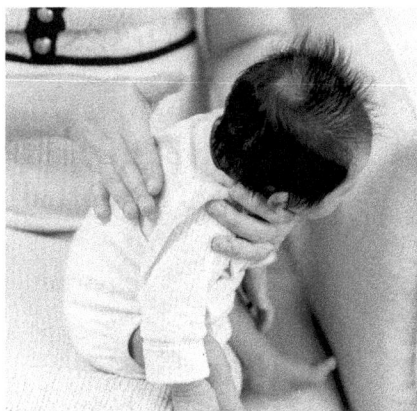

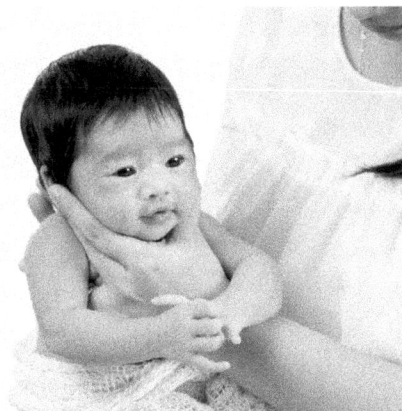

actually involves acupressure for the vagal nerve. This is best done with your baby sitting on your lap. Cup the lower face with the chin resting in the curve of your thumb and index finger. Find the sweet spot for your baby's digestive tract so it does not compress into the stomach, and gently pat the back to release air. Activating the vagal nerve helps relax the whole of the digestive system.

Body Contact

Reasons to spend time doing skin contact, body wearing, prone positioning:
- Skin-to-skin warmth helps the circulation and temperature regulation mature
- Gentle pressure on the belly side helps relax organs & blood vessels
- Autonomic nervous system regulation promotes resiliency
- A great position to get ready for tummy time
- Relieves pressure off the back of the skull to help with head shape
- Bonding and connecting emotionally and spiritually with your baby

Chest to chest skin contact

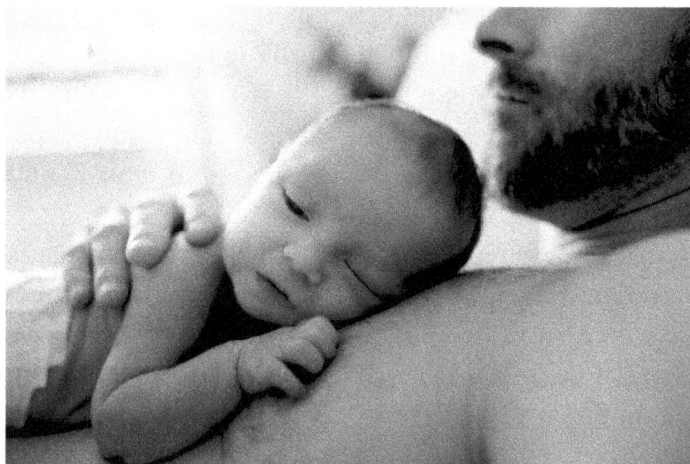

Body wearing

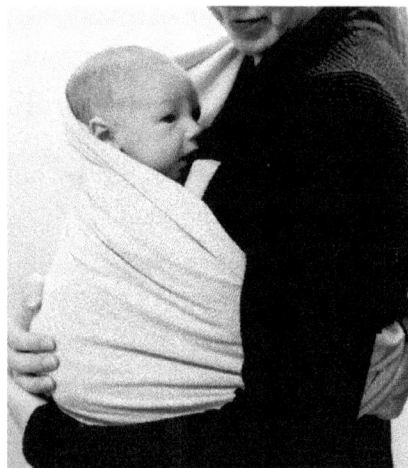

Sloth positioning

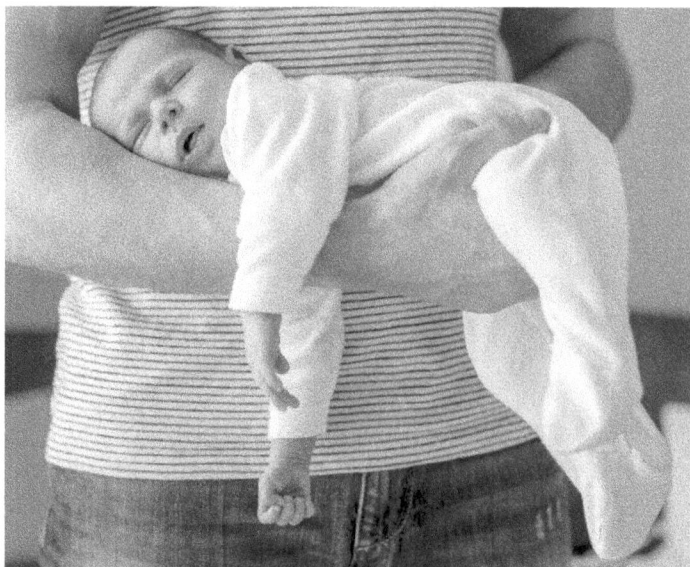

Additional reasons to do sloth positioning (also known as football hold):

- Stretches important nerves in the spine
- Helps rib cage to fully expand so heart and lungs adjust out of the womb
- Gentle pressure into belly organs helps relax digestion for better colic relief.

Side-lying holding

We have found a side-lying hold is a very effective, less-stressful way to help stretch a consistent head tilt to one side (torticollis). Hold your baby on the side the head tips towards. Nestle your arm in the curve of the side of the neck (as seen in the photo). Hold their hips to stabilize their body from turning. Gently, so gently, slowly raise your elbow to lift their head upward, stretching the shortened side of the neck. Hold as long as your baby tolerates, anywhere from 10 seconds to 5 minutes. Repeat several times a day. Remember, slow and steady movement. Match the resistance of their muscles. The support you give their body will make neck stretches less distressing than trying to stretch their neck when they lay on their back.

Reasons to do this:

- Easiest and less distressing way to stretch tight neck side for torticollis
- Stretches not just the neck but the whole side of the body
- Helps neck and vision work together for a sense of "middle"
- Be sure to practice holding on both sides to balance eye focus

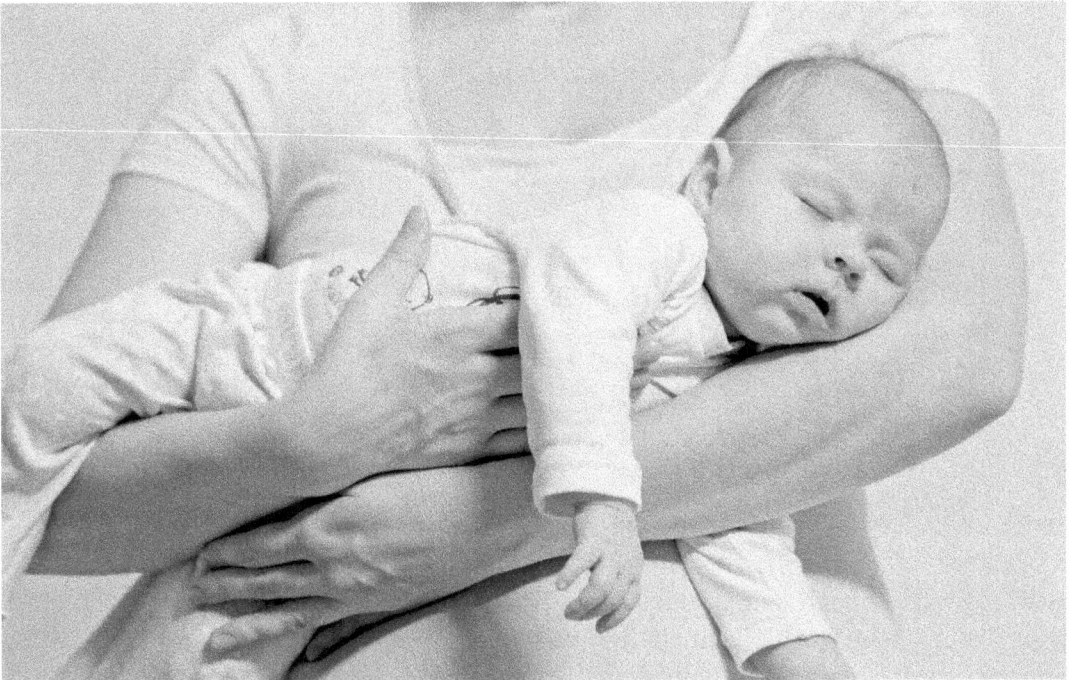

Play and Lay Positions

Lay or Play in Side Lying

Side lying is an often over looked position for play during awake and alert times with your baby. Having head, neck, and spine align is one of the benefits while at the same time relieving any potential pressure spots on the skull.

This play and lay position is also a non-stressful way to stretch a shortened neck.

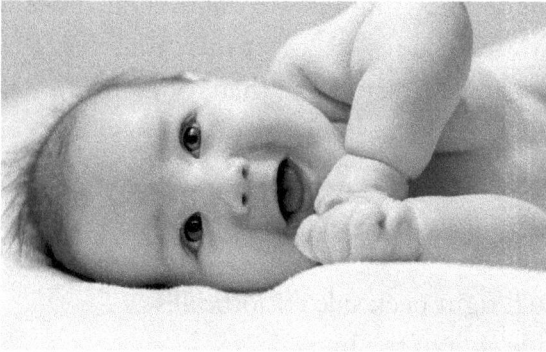

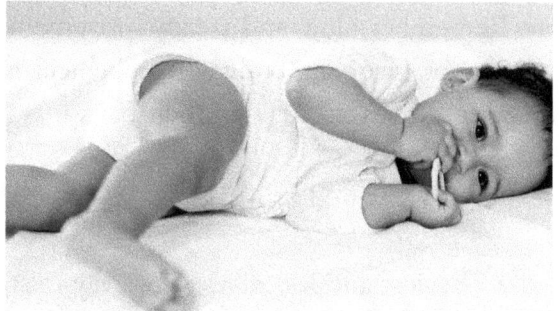

As their neck and shoulder muscles becomes stronger, they begin to redistribute pressure on the skull more evenly.

Lap Supported

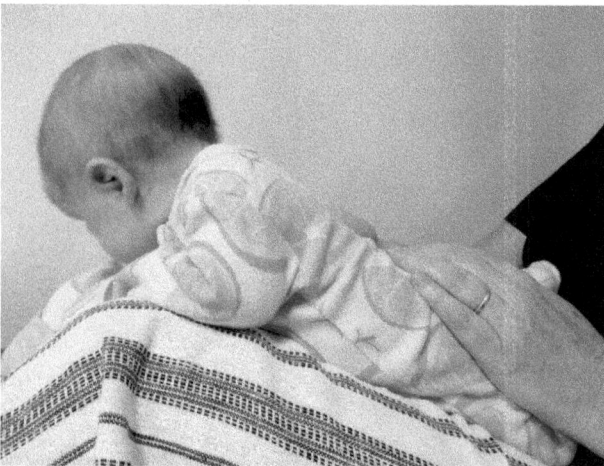

- Provides a comfy surface for needed pressure for belly organs while provide a back massage, without the full weight of gravity.
- Builds readiness for good tummy time.
- Stretches organs and major blood vessels in the belly and chest.
- Strengthens back and neck muscles in a more gradual manner.
- Semi upright helps relieve gas bubbles for a burp and reduces reflux.
- Great for helping create toots for gas relief.

Resting on the couch with your knees bent, having your baby semi-reclined in such a manner. Tummy makes full contact with your thighs. Reasons this play position is helpful:

Body Supported

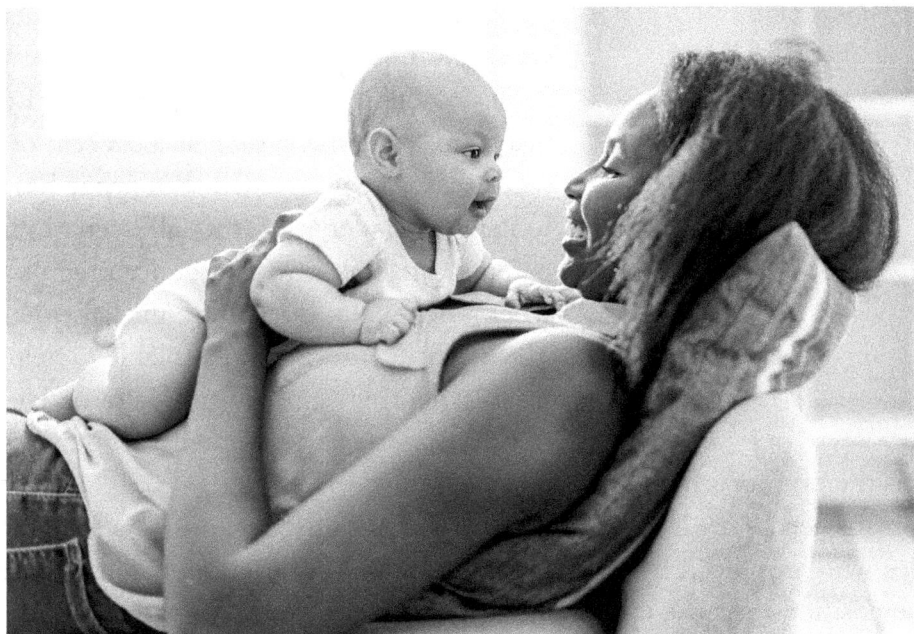

Pressure of tummy into mommy's belly is comforting. Face-to-face can reduce the stress of raising head up. The angle of incline can be changed to match baby's ability to raise self.

Parent-guided Yoga Pose

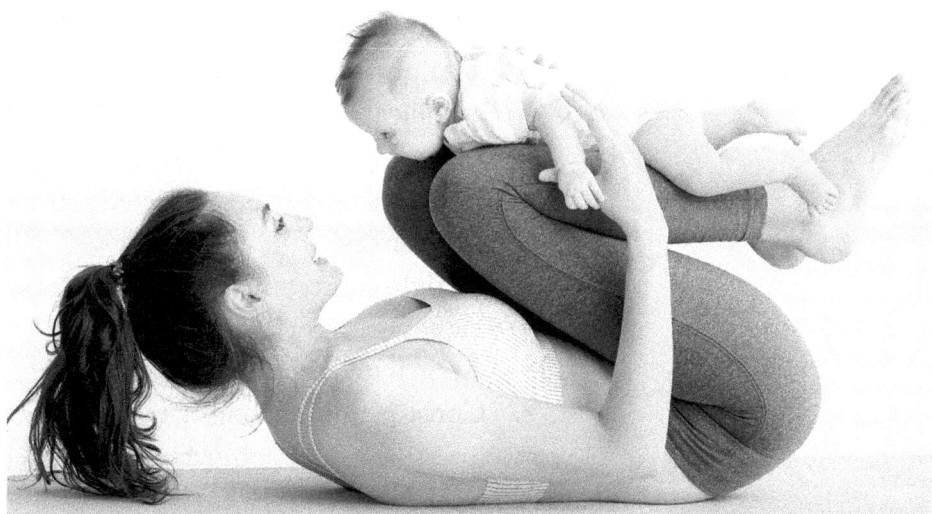

The parent becomes the floor in such a pose, but the weight of their adult legs helps counter the full weight of gravity. Add in the bonus effect of face-to-face connection for bonding and eye contact, mommies can also work on their post-partum exercises.

Belly on the Floor

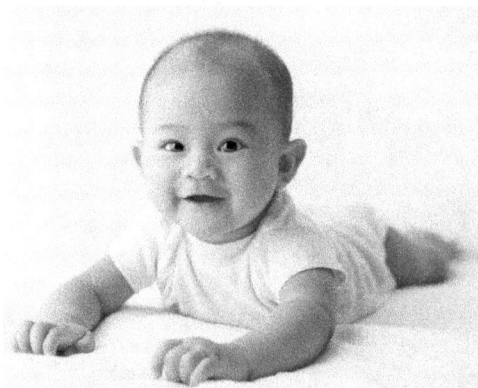

Information on baby development now stress the importance of spending equal time on bellies to being placed on their backs. Less time placed in "containers" such as a car seat or bouncy seat is also recommended. But what has seemed to happen is a "one-size-fits-all" scenario in which parents can be left to feel guilty or hide the fact when their baby doesn't fit into the new rules. There is little information available to help parents troubleshooting or navigate alternatives when tummy time is not tolerated or hours in a sling seat swing is the only soother.

Humans need more information to ward off negative feelings or judgments. Many, many babies who have been brought to me in such a scenario and parents confess they avoid prone positions because it makes their baby cry and fuss. No parent enjoys making their baby cry. Here are common discoveries through bodywork we see causing discomfort or intolerance of lying flat on tummies, listed in the order of most common:

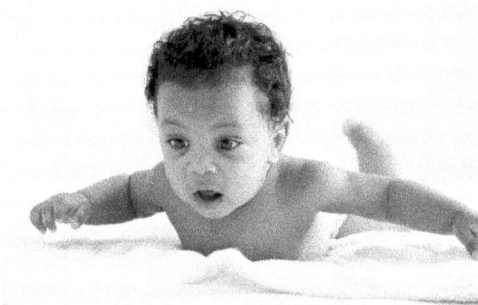

- The deep front line fascia band prevents a full guppy pose (arching backward under their own power)
- A tight and restricted remnant of the umbilical cord, behind the belly button and extending up into the liver
- Extremely tight and restricted psoas muscles (hip flexors)
- A tight, restricted, often twisted respiratory diaphragm and lower ribs
- An irritated esophagus from reflux
- Constipation and tight tissues surrounding intestines; tight sphincters

If your baby struggles to be soothed, does not tolerate recommended positioning, or has body and head asymmetries, they are indicating to you that Bodywork could be beneficial

Summary

These methods were described as user-friendly as possible so you can practice them easily. The knowledge comes from twenty-five years of fusing these methods into daily clinical practice and then teaching family after family how to help things continue at home for long-term health and wellness. Based upon thousands of patient encounters, the outcomes have been consistently positive for otherwise healthy babies needing help adjusting.'

These methods are not only enjoyable and interactive, but they also foster a strong bond between you and your baby. They are specifically designed to be non-invasive, ensuring that you and your baby can engage in them without stress or guilt. Remember, bodywork is a tool to help us understand your baby's needs and assist them in self-correcting their struggles, all in a gentle and respectful manner.

It's crucial to understand that bodywork is not a substitute for primary healthcare. However, a trained practitioner in these (or other) methods can serve as a valuable guide. This ensures that you are never alone in your baby's health and wellness journey. Bodywork experiences can provide you with the support and knowledge to recognize when further medical referral may be necessary for your baby's well-being.

These methods make up the collection called Bodywork for Babies:
- CranioSacral Therapy (CST)*
- Visceral maneuvers or manipulation
- Lympho-fascia and lymphatic fluid mobilization
- Myofascial release methods
- Acupressure

*It is recommended that CST be the fundamental knowledge for the kind of perfect touch for working with babies. Practitioners may have other skill sets in different methods. Still, CST's non-invasive, gentle, and safe touch lets parents know that all other methods follow suit. A practitioner without CST training may touch too heavily, too aggressively, and too much in control of tissues. CST is a practice of being in the right spots to help with self-correction.

Bodywork for Babies highlights skill sets but not a particular profession. Anyone with a professional license to touch therapeutically can become trained. *Bodywork for Babies* is about helping babies self-correct, a concept unique to these methods. This is done with helping hands (or fingertips) placed on the "just right spot."

Parents are great resources for other parents, but finding someone in your community may be challenging without a personal referral. The following pages offer resources of international therapist directories to guide you, the savvy healthcare consumer, in finding a qualified person to work with you and your baby.

Resources

This resource guide is meant to empower you with knowledge to help your baby feel better within their tiny bodies. If you feel the need to seek professional help, there are some things to keep in mind. Bodywork methods are not owned by any specific profession. Different professionals can advertise and engage in bodywork practices for babies. This includes occupational therapists, physical therapists, massage therapists, chiropractors, osteopathic physicians, nurses, and others. There is a large variety of training sources for bodywork. From formal instruction by experts to informal and casual learning, skill sets range from novice to sage experts.

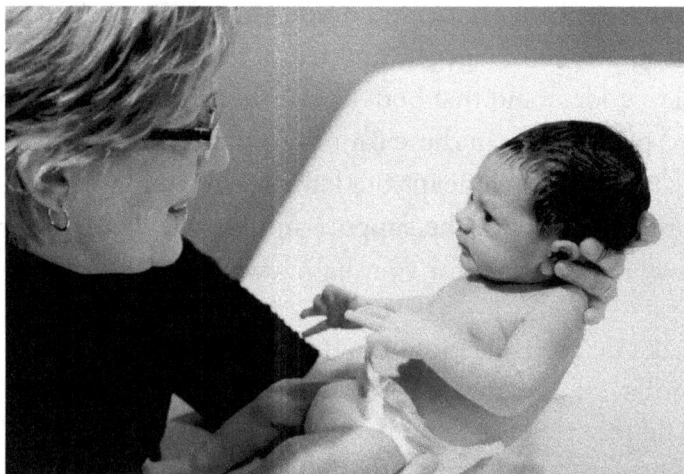

Consider asking your potential bodyworker these questions:

1. What were your training qualifications for infant bodywork methods?
2. What institute did you train for CranioSacral Therapy, visceral manipulation, or lymphatic drainage?
3. How many classes have you attended, and were they in-person or online?
4. What method guides the level of touch pressure you use?
5. Does the training method used have peer review or a certification process? (Certification offers assurance that training is from the original source, and raises public safety in reliable services that pass peer-testing).
6. Is there an established directory from the training institute(s) to inform the public of the level of such training?

The author's bias is toward four Institutes, all promoting high standards for student education while promoting advanced levels of training to usher practitioners toward expert skill sets.

International Alliance of Healthcare Educators

1. Upledger Institute International
    Original source of CranioSacral Therapy and somato-emotional release

2. Barral Institute International
    Original source for visceral manipulation; neuro-manipulation

3. D'Ambrogio Institute
    An osteopathic approach to total body balancing

4. The Chikly Health Institute
    Lymphatic and Lympho-fascia Drainage; Brain Curriculum

Doctors of osteopathy will have specific manual medicine training during the course of the medical school education. Chiropractors will have post-graduate training exclusive for pediatric practice. Other professional therapists have sought training worldwide from the above-mentioned institutes for over forty years.

A worldwide network of innovative and progressive-thinking therapists, created by John Matthew Upledger, gives clients a resource to find local care.

International Alliance of Healthcare Practitioners
11211 Prosperity Farms Road, Suite D-325
Palm Beach Gardens, FL 33410-3487
Toll free: 800-311-9204
website: https://www.iahp.com/

FIND A PRACTITIONER makes it easy to locate a practitioner in your area. An *advanced* search can help you locate someone with specialty training in pediatrics. Also, the practitioner's license helps you understand their professional approach. The background of the practitioner also cues you to their depth-of-knowledge of pediatric care.

Both Upledger and Barral Institutes have formal certification and diplomat levels.

Chikly Health Institute (CHI) approved courses are eligible to be listed in their online directory. This directory lists attendance, but does warrant the quality of skills or services. They also provide certification level training.

INDEX

www.ingramcontent.com/pod-product-compliance
Lightning Source LLC
Chambersburg PA
CBHW081410270326
41931CB00016B/3433